DEPARTMENT OF HEALTH

On the State of
THE PUBLIC HEALTH

to be ret   re

THE ANNUAL REPORT OF
THE CHIEF MEDICAL OFFICER OF
THE DEPARTMENT OF HEALTH
FOR THE YEAR 1994

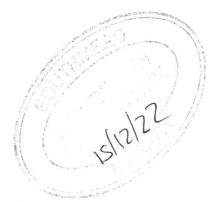

15/12/22

LONDON

D0277431

ISBN 0 11 321910 5

CONTENTS

INTRODUCTION   1

EXECUTIVE SUMMARY   12

1. VITAL STATISTICS   41
    (a) Population size   41
    (b) Age and sex structure of the resident population   41
    (c) Fertility statistics - aspects of relevance for health care   41
    (d) Mortality   46
    (e) Prevalence of disease in the community   48
    (f) Infant and perinatal mortality   52
    (g) Trends in cancer incidence and mortality   53
    (h) Trends in reporting congenital malformations   54
    (i) Appendix Tables and their content (pages 239-250)   55

2. THE NATION'S HEALTH   59
    (a) Public health in England   59
    (b) Regional perspective   60
    (c) Inter-Departmental Group on Public Health   63
    (d) Urban and rural differences in health   63
    (e) Variations in health   64
    (f) Substance misuse   65
    (g) Nutrition   69
    (h) Health of people in later life   70
    (i) Health of black and ethnic minorities   71
    (j) Health of men   72
    (k) Health of adolescents   74

3. THE STRATEGY FOR HEALTH   76
    (a) Introduction   76
    (b) Key areas and targets   77
         (i)   Coronary heart disease and stroke   77
         (ii)   Cancers   78
         (iii) Mental illness   79
         (iv)   HIV/AIDS and sexual health   80
         (v)   Accidents   81
    (c) Implementation   83
         (i)   Priorities for the NHS   83
         (ii)   Local health alliances   85
         (iii) Healthy settings   85
         (iv)   Inter-Departmental co-operation   86
    (d) The way ahead   86

4. HEALTH IN THE WORKPLACE   88
    (a) Introduction   88
    (b) Occupational health today   89
         (i)   The changing industrial base and pattern of employment   89
         (ii)   Societal changes and public expectations   90
         (iii) International influences   90
    (c) What is occupational health?   90
         (i)   The effect of work on health   91

		(ii)	The effect of health on work	91
		(iii)	Health promotion	91
	(d)	Legislative and organisational framework		92
	(e)	Information about occupational ill-health		93
	(f)	Main occupational health hazards, diseases and disorders		97
		(i)	Chemical risks and diseases	98
		(ii)	Physical risks and diseases	106
		(iii)	Biological hazards and diseases	112
		(iv)	Work-related psychosocial risks and ill-health	115
		(v)	Rural issues	116
	(g)	Effects of health on work		118
	(h)	Health promotion		119
	(i)	Occupational health services		120
	(j)	Ethics and confidentiality		120
	(k)	Health of NHS staff		121
	(l)	Responsibilities and training		122
	(m)	Audit in occupational health		122
	(n)	Research		123
	(o)	Future developments and emerging issues		124
		(i)	Strategic health risk reviews	124
		(ii)	Reproductive health	125
		(iii)	Genetic screening	125
		(iv)	Environmental issues	125
		(v)	International issues	126
		(vi)	The way ahead	126
5.	HEALTH CARE			128
	(a)	Needs, effectiveness and outcomes		128
		(i)	Health needs assessment	128
		(ii)	Basic sources of information	128
		(iii)	National confidential enquiries	129
		(iv)	Quality of service and effectiveness of care	130
		(v)	National Casemix Office and NHS Centre for Coding and Classification	130
		(vi)	Clinical outcomes	132
	(b)	Primary health care		133
		(i)	Organisation of primary care	133
		(ii)	Prescribing	135
		(iii)	Professional development	136
		(iv)	The way ahead	136
	(c)	Hospital services		137
		(i)	Specialised services	137
		(ii)	Cancer	137
		(iii)	Thromboprophylaxis	137
		(iv)	Minimal access surgery	138
		(v)	Osteoporosis	138
		(vi)	Transplantation	139
	(d)	Diabetes mellitus		140
	(e)	Asthma		140
	(f)	Complementary medicine		141
	(g)	Mental health		141
		(i)	Mental health and primary care	141
		(ii)	Occupational mental health	142
		(iii)	Confidential Inquiry into Homicides and Suicides	142

	(iv)	Services for people with severe mental illness	143
	(v)	Services for mentally disordered offenders	144
	(vi)	Mental health legislation	145
(h)		Maternity and child health services	146
	(i)	Implementation of 'Changing Childbirth'	146
	(ii)	Confidential Enquiries into Maternal Deaths	146
	(iii)	Folic acid and prevention of neural tube defects	147
	(iv)	Human Fertilisation and Embryology Authority	147
	(v)	Sudden infant death syndrome	148
	(vi)	Prophylaxis of vitamin K deficiency bleeding in infants	148
	(vii)	Retinopathy of prematurity	149
	(viii)	Paediatric intensive care	150
	(ix)	Confidential Enquiry into Stillbirths and Deaths in Infancy	150
	(x)	Congenital malformations	151
	(xi)	Gene Therapy Advisory Committee	152
	(xii)	Code of practice on special education needs and circulars on 'Pupils with problems'	152
(i)		Learning disabilities	154
(j)		Disability and rehabilitation	155
(k)		Prison health care	155
(l)		London Implementation Group	156

6.		COMMUNICABLE DISEASES	159
(a)		HIV infection and AIDS	159
(b)		Other sexually transmitted diseases	167
(c)		Immunisation	171
(d)		Viral hepatitis	179
(e)		Influenza	182
(f)		Tuberculosis	183
(g)		Plague	183
(h)		Necrotising fasciitis	184
(i)		Antibiotic resistance and hospital-acquired infection	185
(j)		Foodborne and waterborne diseases	185
(k)		Travel-related disease	189

7.		ENVIRONMENTAL HEALTH AND TOXICOLOGY	192
(a)		Chemical and physical agents in the environment	192
	(i)	Small Area Health Statistics Unit	192
	(ii)	Air pollution	192
	(iii)	Institute for Environment and Health	194
	(iv)	Committee on Medical Aspects of Radiation in the Environment	194
	(v)	Environment and health	194
	(vi)	Surveillance of diseases possibly due to non-infectious environmental hazards	195
(b)		Toxicological safety	196
	(i)	Food chemical hazards	196
	(ii)	Food carcinogen prioritisation	197
	(iii)	Peanut anaphylaxis	197
	(iv)	Traditional remedies	197
	(v)	The Advisory Committee on Novel Foods and Processes	198
	(vi)	Genetically modified food plants	198
	(vii)	Fat replacers	198

	(viii)	Man-made mineral fibres	199
	(ix)	Organization for Economic Co-operation and Development guidelines for testing chemicals for toxicity	199
	(x)	Pesticides	199
	(xi)	Veterinary drugs	200
8.	**MEDICAL EDUCATION, TRAINING AND STAFFING**		**202**
	(a)	Junior doctors' hours	202
	(b)	'Achieving a Balance' and the Advisory Group on Medical and Dental Education, Training and Staffing	203
	(c)	Medical Manpower Standing Advisory Committee	204
	(d)	Equal opportunities for doctors	204
	(e)	Part-time consultants scheme	205
	(f)	New career structure for doctors in child health	206
	(g)	Postgraduate, continuing and specialist medical education	206
	(h)	Medical (Professional Performance) Bill	208
	(i)	Undergraduate medical and dental education	208
	(j)	Doctors' performance	209
	(k)	Locum doctors	209
9.	**OTHER TOPICS OF INTEREST IN 1994**		**210**
	(a)	Medicines Control Agency	210
		(i) Role and performance	210
		(ii) Control of UK clinical trials	210
		(iii) Legal reclassification of medicinal products	211
		(iv) Pharmaceutical developments in the European Community	211
	(b)	European Medicines Evaluation Agency	212
	(c)	Medical Devices Agency	213
	(d)	National Blood Authority	215
	(e)	National Biological Standards Board	215
	(f)	National Radiological Protection Board	216
	(g)	United Kingdom Transplant Support Service Agency	218
	(h)	Microbiological Research Authority	219
	(i)	Creutzfeldt-Jakob Disease Surveillance Unit	219
	(j)	Bioethics	219
		(i) Local Research Ethics Committees	219
		(ii) Bioethics in Europe	221
		(iii) Genetic screening	221
		(iv) Draft guidance on confidentiality	221
		(v) House of Lords Select Committee in Medical Ethics	222
	(k)	Research and development	222
		(i) White Paper on Science, Engineering and Technology	222
		(ii) Research for health	223
		(iii) Developments in the NHS research and development programme	223
	(l)	Dental health	224
		(i) Dental health of the nation	224
		(ii) General dental services	225
		(iii) Community dental services	226
		(iv) Hospital dental services	227
		(v) Continuing education and training for dentists	227
		(vi) Dental research	228

10. INTERNATIONAL HEALTH   229
  (a) England, Europe and health   229
  (b) The European Community   229
      (i)   The Council of Health Ministers   229
      (ii)   EC/WHO/Council of Europe   230
      (iii) European Economic Area   230
      (iv)   Free movement of people   230
      (v)   Channel Tunnel and port health checks   231
      (vi)   Draft Directive on Data Protection   231
      (vii) Smoking   231
      (viii) Elderly and disabled people   232
      (ix)   AIDS and HIV infection   232
      (x)   Research and information technology   232
      (xi)   Food safety   233
      (xii) Medical Devices Directives   233
  (c) Relations with Central and Eastern Europe   234
  (d) Council of Europe   235
  (e) Organization for Economic Co-operation and Development   235
  (f) The Commonwealth   236
  (g) World Health Organization   236
      (i)   European Regional Committee   236
      (ii)   Executive Board   237
      (iii) World Health Assembly   237

APPENDIX   239

INTRODUCTION

Rt Hon Stephen Dorrell MP
Secretary of State for Health

Sir,

I have pleasure in submitting my Report on the State of the Public Health for 1994, together with some comments on the more important developments and events in the first half of 1995. This Report is the 137th of the series which began in 1858.

I am pleased to report that there were considerable improvements in health over the year: infant mortality is at the lowest recorded rate. Infectious diseases continue to cause concern; however, the measles/rubella immunisation campaign in November to prevent a predicted epidemic of measles was a great success. Much progress was made towards more integrated working to maintain the public health, and for more efficient communications between all those involved. The White Paper *The Health of the Nation: a strategy for health in England*[1] continues to provide an important impetus for improving health. Launched in July 1992, it has been taken up with vigour by a wide range of organisations. Encouraging progress has been made towards most of the targets set although, as is pointed out in this Report, some targets present particular challenges.

As I discussed last year, this Report is not simply a document of record, but must also try to interpret and to explain changes in those factors that are known to influence and to determine health, and should identify areas where improvements could be made. In previous years, I have highlighted some issues for special mention, with the intention that they would be followed up in subsequent Reports. Topics identified in earlier years have been acted on and progress is discussed in this Report. Four key issues are identified for broader discussion during the coming year: health in the workplace, equity and equality, food poisoning, and drug and solvent misuse. It is hoped that over the next year these four topics will stimulate interest, and I shall report back on these areas in next year's Report.

I wish to acknowledge the help and support given to me by numerous colleagues in the Department of Health and the Office of Population Censuses and Surveys in the preparation of this Report, and the assistance of Her Majesty's Stationery Office, Norwich, which arranged the printing and publication.

I am, Sir,
Your obedient servant

Kenneth C Calman

September 1995

LONG TERM STRATEGIC AIMS

Previous Reports[2,3] set out a series of long-term strategic aims which also underpin the content of this Report:

- To promote efforts to ensure health for all;

- To achieve the targets in the strategy for health;

- To involve patients and the public in choices and decision-making;

- To establish an effective intelligence and information system for public health and clinical practice;

- To ensure a health service based on an assessment of health needs, quality of care and effectiveness of outcome; *and*

- To provide a highly professional team of staff with strong education, research and ethical standards.

These six points continue to provide the strategic direction and intent of the Report.

HEALTH IN ENGLAND IN 1994

During the period of this Report there have been a number of important improvements in health. The infant mortality rate at 6.1 per 1,000 live births is the lowest ever, and since 1993 there has been a 17% fall in malformed live births to 69.2 per 10,000 live births. Conceptions under the age of 16 years dropped in 1992 to 8.4 per 1,000 girls aged 13-15 years, a very encouraging fall from the 1991 figure of 9.3. Post-neonatal mortality dropped by 53% in the period 1988-94 and is now at 2.0 per 1,000 live births. There has been a 71% reduction in post-neonatal sudden infant deaths over the same period.

Of particular significance was the measles/rubella immunisation campaign in November; there was an overall 92% uptake among a target population of 7.17 million children, and since the beginning of 1995 there have been very few cases of confirmed measles. This campaign was a major success and we will continue to work towards eliminating measles in this country. Other infectious diseases were of concern, notably necrotising fasciitis in February, and the possibility of the plague in September. In the early months of 1995, there was an outbreak of Ebola virus infection in Zaire. The level of food poisoning in this country continues to rise and this is discussed in more detail on page 8.

In last year's Report[4], I raised the issue of changing patterns of infectious diseases, and emphasised the need to be vigilant and to have in place mechanisms to deal with potential outbreaks. During the year, surveillance systems and control mechanisms became fully operative and there was excellent co-operation between Government Departments and the Public Health

Laboratory Service (PHLS). Experience during 1994 has shown how necessary this is, and it is essential that we retain the capacity to react swiftly to potential threats to health.

For this reason it has been important to set up improved methods of communication with doctors and other health and environmental health professionals. This has involved setting up an electronic communication system, which will be improved and developed over the next few years. It has proved invaluable in dealing with public health incidents over the last year. In addition, the quarterly *CMO's Update* has replaced many of the CMO Letters previously used to inform doctors about specific issues, and has been shown to be a most useful medium. Coupled with the development of the national Public Health Network, mechanisms for continuing to improve the public health function are now in place and will be regularly updated.

In terms of clinical practice, the main thrust has been to ensure the continuing development of programmes to improve outcomes. The culture of evidence-based clinical practice with an emphasis on effectiveness and appropriateness is now flourishing in the National Health Service (NHS). There are close links between this programme, clinical audit, research and development initiatives, and the professional organisations. This work is co-ordinated by the Clinical Outcomes Group (COG) chaired jointly by the Chief Nursing Officer and myself. One example of this work was the report of an Expert Advisory Group on Cancer Services to the Chief Medical Officers of England and Wales, setting out a framework for change and improvement of services to patients[5]. A central feature of this process is the development, by the professions, of clinical guidelines to maintain and improve standards of care and outcome indicators to assess achievement, thus improving clinical outcomes through good clinical practice.

THE STRATEGY FOR HEALTH

The third anniversary of the publication of the Health of the Nation White Paper[1] was marked on 3 July 1995 with a major conference to launch the Health of the Young Nation - a new initiative within the Health of the Nation framework which picks up on issues which were set out in the special chapter of my Report for 1993[6].

We shall also be publishing a second report on progress on Health of the Nation; I am delighted to say that we are moving in the right direction in most areas. Statistics for 1994 indicate reductions on 1993 levels for 10 of the 11 mortality targets. Although single-year changes must be viewed with caution, encouraging falls of above 5% have occurred for coronary heart disease (CHD), stroke, accidents and suicide. It is also particularly pleasing to see how far the concept of joint working has spread in such a relatively short time; other Government Departments are making important contributions in their various policy areas, and the Alliance Award Scheme entries have shown innumerable examples of health promotion projects involving health authorities, voluntary organisations and other groups as well as the health services. With the development of my Health Challenge into a number of targeted Health Challenges, we are also drawing businesses into partnerships for health promotion. Challenges remain in the targets for reduction of obesity, teenage cigarette smoking and suicide in young men. In the last few months, we have published a document for hospital doctors to encourage their participation in achieving Health of the Nation targets[7].

Part of the task of the Working Group I chair has been to look in detail at the variations in health relevant to the NHS for the five key areas in the strategy for health. This work is proceeding and will be completed in the Autumn of 1995. The issues of equity and equality which arise from this work are discussed on page 7.

Looking further afield, we are also involved in the development of a European network for health promotion in the workplace. This is a particularly exciting development; there is tremendous scope for spreading healthy messages and for engaging employers and employees - both corporately and as individuals - in activities to improve health. This ties in well with our own initiative to set up a team to support and encourage the formation of partnerships between businesses for workplace health promotion.

PROGRESS ON ACTION POINTS IN PREVIOUS REPORTS

Each year, topics which have been highlighted in previous Reports are reviewed and any action noted.

Progress on topics raised in 1991

The health of ethnic minorities remains a high priority to the Department and is an important consideration in the development of health policy. The Ethnic Health Unit in Leeds is now fully operational. A better understanding of the use of NHS services by people from ethnic minorities will be available in the future with the inclusion from 1 April 1995 of ethnic monitoring as part of the Contract Minimum Data Set for inpatient and day cases. Through this information, purchasers and providers will be able to identify gaps in service provision and ascertain particular needs for secondary care. Ethnic monitoring of the NHS workforce has also been introduced and will enable progress towards the goal of equal opportunities, to be monitored by the NHS Executive.

The changes in *medical education* within medical schools in response to the General Medical Council's report *Tomorrow's doctors*[8] are progressing well, with good examples of innovative approaches to changing the curriculum. The changes in postgraduate medical education following the report, *Hospital doctors: training for the future*[9], are also progressing well. The medical Royal Colleges are developing their programmes of continuing professional education and development. The early part of 1995 has seen significant progress on a number of issues, in particular the publication of the reports[10] of the working groups set up to consider in detail the implications of *Hospital doctors: training for the future*[9]. The groups considered the implications for overseas doctors, general medical practice, and academic and research medicine of the introduction

4

of a unified training grade. The publication of the reports, all of which are consultation documents, gives the profession at large the opportunity to contribute to setting the direction for the development of postgraduate medical education in the United Kingdom (UK) for the future.

The COG is co-ordinating work on *clinical audit* and is involved in the broader issues of clinical guidelines and outcomes assessment. A great deal of work is in progress within the NHS Executive and the professions.

Over the past year the results of a major survey carried out in England and Wales in 1993 on all cases of *tuberculosis* have started to become available, and should provide a most useful basis for considering future plans to control this infection.

Progress on topics identified in 1992

Men's health issues are increasingly being discussed and several major conferences on the topic have been arranged. Nevertheless, men may still delay before seeking advice and treatment, and we still have a long way to go in improving the health of men.

Cigarette smoking remains the largest preventable cause of death and ill-health in this country. In spite of this knowledge, people continue to smoke in large numbers; 28% of adults in England are regular smokers. The uptake of cigarette smoking is largely determined in the teenage years and surveys have established that nearly 70% of 15-year-olds have tried cigarette smoking at some time. Progress towards achieving the Health of the Nation target for smoking prevalence among young people has been disappointing, and contrasts with the steady decline in adult smoking prevalence (see page 65). This discrepancy will require more work and innovative thinking; greater attention may need to be paid to smoking cessation programmes. March 1994 saw the setting up of the Scientific Committee on Tobacco and Health (SCOTH), which reports directly to me on scientific and behavioural aspects of tobacco use. Its November meeting was devoted to smoking and young people in order to gain better understanding of the factors that influence young people to smoke, and to inform wider Departmental thinking on future Health of the Nation target developments. Smoking among young people is a difficult area and significant progress towards the Government's target to reduce smoking prevalence in this group will depend on a number of factors - not least by reducing cigarette smoking prevalence in adults and by influencing public opinion to reduce the social acceptability of the smoking habit.

The provision of services to meet the needs of *mentally disordered offenders* remains a high priority for the NHS. The number of beds available for treatment in medium security conditions has increased sharply so that, by the end of 1996, some 2,000 beds (including beds aimed at meeting the need for longer term care), should be available to the NHS, compared with 1,100 beds available in 1994. Transfers of patients from prison to inpatient care has continued at a high level, with 792 patients being transferred in 1994 (Home Office: provisional data). Changes in the funding and organisation of high security services announced recently[11] will over time greatly improve the services available to all patients who need treatment in such conditions.

A major report was published in June 1995[12] on the problems associated with *verocytotoxin-producing Escherichia coli (VTEC)* and a number of recommendations made as to its control. A specific recommendation on the use of unpasteurised milk has been made, and I have warned vulnerable sections of the public about the dangers of drinking raw milk[13].

Progress on topics identified in 1993

There has been increasing interest in the *health of adolescents* following the publication of the Report for 1993[6]. The Department of Health (DH) launched an initiative to target young people as part of the Health of the Nation strategy at a conference on 3 July 1995. This initiative will interpret health broadly, and will emphasise the pan-Government nature of the initiative. The Department's Central Research and Development Committee Advisory Group on Mother and Child Health will report shortly. Among the priorities are recommendations relevant to NHS provision for adolescents. From 1996, the DH centrally commissioned research programme will be funding research on behavioural change and health promotion, part of which will be concerned with adolescent behaviour. Preparation for this includes a review of effectiveness of health promotion interventions for adolescents across the Health of the Nation key areas. DH has also given priority to adolescent mental health; with the then Department for Education (DFE) it published jointly a handbook on child and adolescent mental health services (CAMHS) in April 1995[14]. This built on the findings of a national review of services for the mental health of children and young people, and was followed by the report of a thematic view of CAMHS by the NHS Health Advisory Service.

Much work continues concerning *asthma*, particularly in relation to air quality. Several important reports will be published in the next few months. Later in 1995, DH and the Department of the Environment, in association with the Institute for Environment and Health and the National Asthma Campaign, will host a conference in London. Its purpose is to provide a balanced view of what is known about the causes of asthma and what can be done to alleviate its effects and prevent new cases.

Genetic factors and disease were raised in last year's Report to indicate their importance for health and health care. A large number of developments have occurred, and these are discussed on page 152.

Last year I raised the *changing patterns of infectious disease* as a topic of particular importance and, on page 2, I have already described some of the events which occurred over the year. In addition, in May 1995 the World Health Assembly passed a resolution to develop strategies to improve the recognition of, and response to, new, emerging, and re-emerging infectious diseases in a manner sustainable by all countries.

NEW ISSUES IDENTIFIED DURING 1994

Each year a small number of issues will be identified as topics of particular importance, to be followed up in subsequent Reports. It should be recognised that the actions needed to ensure progress on these topics may be the responsibility of a wide range of organisations and individuals.

One general issue I wish to raise before outlining four major areas for attention this year concerns the increasing importance of ethical dimensions to health and health care. The values upon which such ethical decisions are made are crucial in the multicultural context of England today. The issues raised - whether they be about confidentiality, resource allocation, euthanasia, research, autonomy, access to health care, inequalities, reproductive health, or one of many others - need wide discussion. This debate is necessary to clarify thinking and to assist in making decisions about patients or communities in which there is real uncertainty and for which there may be no 'right' answer. Judgment is difficult, as was recognised by Hippocrates centuries ago - "Life is short, the art long, the occasion fleeting; experience fallacious and judgment difficult".

Health in the workplace

The special chapter in this year's Report outlines some of the important effects of work on health, the effects of health on work, and the value of health promotion in the workplace. Risks from chemicals, radiation and other physical agents, and from biological factors are outlined. Risk assessment and management are highlighted. In particular, it emphasises the burden of work-related ill-health and associated costs to industry, and to the country. The chapter makes a special mention of mental health problems at work related to stress and employment issues. It notes the importance of occupational health services, and points to ways to improve health at work. The next year should see a number of initiatives in this area, many targeted at small and medium-sized companies. Co-operation in the form of partnerships between employers and employees, the Confederation of British Industry, trade unions and many others will be necessary if real improvements are to be made.

Equity and equality

There is increasing interest in variations in health and health care and the inequities and inequalities which can occur. Over the past year a number of reports have highlighted these variations, which are well recognised and have been for a long time. The accurate recording of information on health, begun in the early 19th century, made such differences apparent - and they still exist.

Health is determined by a number of factors including biological and genetic factors, lifestyle and behaviour, the environment (including communicable diseases), social and economic factors, and health services. In all of these, the concepts of equity and equality are important and the variations in health and health care which exist may be related to any of them - either alone or, more frequently, in combination. The term 'variations' is essentially neutral and is used to describe factual information about health and health care. However, the words 'equity' and 'equality' are often used interchangeably despite important distinctions between them. Equity is about fairness and justice, and implies that everyone should have an opportunity to attain their full potential for health. Equality, on the other hand, is about comparisons between the level of health, or ability to obtain access to health care, of individuals and communities. Some inequalities may be unavoidable, and therefore generally not considered unfair, while others might be avoided and so considered inequitable. Natural, biological and genetic variations may have unavoidable (though very important) health inequalities related to them. Lifestyle and behaviour patterns chosen by individuals can also result in inequalities in health - for example, cigarette smoking. In some instances health promotion activities, if selectively taken up, may even increase the inequalities - but again this might not be considered inequitable as they are the result of personal choice. However, lifestyle and behaviour that is not freely chosen, and which results in poorer health, might be considered as avoidable and thus inequitable. Health inequalities arising from the level of resources, housing conditions, dangerous working conditions, or exposure to environmental hazards, and which lead to health inequalities, would be examples of these. Inadequate access to health care or other public services might also be inequitable if the cause was avoidable and the result was inequality: such factors might include transport, lack of information, or inaccessibility of information as a result of language difficulties.

The NHS is strongly committed to the concept of equity, which is one of its key principles. Action to tackle some of the inequalities by the NHS is a continuous process. The report of the Variations in Health Sub-group concentrates specifically on action by the NHS that will assist progress in the Health of the Nation key areas. In relation to other determinants of health there will need to be further discussion on the physical environment, a greater understanding of the blocks to taking up healthier lifestyles, and more research on the social and economic factors which underpin such issues. The targeting of resources to those most in need, information provision and personal choice are complementary aspects of improving health.

It is hoped that this brief discussion of the distinction between equity and equality will assist in targeting particularly those inequalities which are avoidable. Dealing with issues of inequality is complex and there are no simple solutions. We need more locally based research projects in this area to help to provide some solutions, and the evaluation of such work needs to be as rigorous as in other branches of health services research.

Food poisoning

Notification of food poisoning continues to rise. In the last three years we have seen the biggest increase in the number of cases notified since the late 1980s. There is no clear explanation for this increase, and it is uncertain whether it represents a rise in the level of illness or a rise in the number of people reporting illness to their doctors. Whichever the reason, it is likely that there is still substantial under-reporting of food poisoning.

A study of human infectious intestinal disease in England is under way, and should improve understanding of the true incidence and causes of food poisoning. Set up in 1993, the study is taking place over three years in 70 general practices in the Medical Research Council (MRC) General Practice Framework.

Laboratory isolations reported to the PHLS reveal differing trends for the main food pathogens. Isolations of *Campylobacter* continue to rise while total isolations of *Salmonella* have been at much the same level since 1989. Isolations of VTEC serogroup 0157 in England and Wales in 1994 have levelled off for the first time in over ten years. Although relatively rare, VTEC infections may result in serious illness, including acute renal failure in children. The recent report of the Advisory Committee on the Microbiological Safety of Food[15] recommends measures to reduce the level of illness and also makes research recommendations to enhance understanding of the ability of these organisms to cause disease. Following publication of the report, and in response to one of the Committee's recommendations, I issued a statement advising people vulnerable to infection not to consume raw milk[13]. The purpose of highlighting foodborne illness is to emphasise the need for everybody who handles foodstuffs - from primary production to the domestic kitchen - to be concerned about food hygiene. Adequate cooking and keeping food under proper temperature control are particularly important. DH has convened a group to study possible links between domestic food handling and foodborne disease.

The Government has been working to make food hygiene regulation more effective and less prescriptive. The implementation of the EC Directive on the Hygiene of Foodstuffs through new food hygiene regulations coming into effect this Autumn has given the opportunity to adopt a risk-related approach based on the principles of hazard analysis and critical control points (HACCP). The Department has been promoting these, and assisting in the training of Environmental Health Officers to ensure they are able to apply the new approach effectively. Another important innovation in the regulation is the requirement, for the first time, for food businesses to supervise and instruct staff in food hygiene matters.

Outbreaks of waterborne infection are relatively uncommon. Towards the end of 1994, the Expert Group chaired by Sir John Badenoch was re-convened to review developments in the understanding of cryptosporidiosis. The group plans to report in late 1995.

Drug and solvent misuse

Drug misuse is a serious and growing problem. Population surveys suggest that among schoolchildren, 3% of 12-13-year-olds and 14% of 14-15-year-olds admit to taking an illegal drug. Numbers of drug addicts notified to the Home Office in the three years from 1990 have increased by over 35%.

The Government has set out a three-year strategy for England, *Tackling Drugs Together*[15], published on 10 May 1995. Related initiatives are in hand in Scotland, Wales and Northern Ireland. The strategy is notable for identifying a set of objectives, to be monitored over the three years, bringing together interdependent action needed across several Government Departments and agencies at local level. Chief Executives of District Health Authorities (DHAs) are tasked this year with setting up local drug action teams including representatives of local authority, health authority, police, probation service and prison service interests.

The strategy includes an emphasis on education and prevention. DH has a key role to play, and there are a number of initiatives underway in support of the overall aims of the strategy. In May, the then DFE sent guidance on drug education and dealing with drug-related incidents to all schools; DFE also made available guidance on approaches to drug education within the curriculum, and advice on drug education resources. The Department for Education and Employment (DFEE) is providing nearly £6 million to support staff training and innovative programmes of drug prevention. The Office for Standards in Education will also play an important role in monitoring implementation in schools and considering the role of the youth service in drug prevention. I welcome the role of the DFEE. In DH, initiatives include:

-   a review of the effectiveness of treatment services for drug misusers. The Task Force set up to oversee this wide-ranging review has commissioned a number of projects to inform its report. This includes one of the largest prospective studies of drug misusers in the world. Its report should be delivered to Ministers in January 1996;

-   a new freephone national drugs helpline offering advice and information to drug misusers and their families and friends;

-   a £1 million grant programme to develop services for young people at risk of drug misuse or at an early stage of drug-taking. The benefits of this programme are being comprehensively evaluated;

-   a review of the key role general practitioners (GPs) can play in the care and treatment of drug misusers when supported by specialist services; *and*

-   development by the Health Education Authority of national anti-drug and solvent publicity campaigns, involving private sector expertise and partnerships.

Some young people also experiment with volatile substance misuse. Since 1985, an average of over 100 people annually have died from solvent abuse: over 70% of them have been under 20 years-of-age and many of them have died on what appears to be their first use. An analysis by St George's Hospital Medical School showed a strong correlation between a significant drop in the number of deaths and the timing of DH's 1992 campaign aimed at parents. Latest figures show a continuing drop in the number of deaths. DH is preparing an inter-Departmental response, including recommendations for further action, on a major report on volatile substance abuse by the Advisory Council on the Misuse of Drugs.

Substance misuse is a major and very serious issue affecting society. The costs are high in personal and community terms. The strategy outlined in *Tackling Drugs Together*[15] set a framework for the way ahead; already there are exciting developments in locally based projects and we need to be able to learn from them, and to try new and innovative ways of tackling this challenge. Like most difficult issues, the causes and solutions are likely to be multi-factorial. For this reason, co-ordination and the sharing of experience will be crucial.

EXECUTIVE SUMMARY

VITAL STATISTICS

Population size

The resident population of England at 30 June 1994 was 48.7 million, a 0.4% increase compared with 1993.

Age and sex structure of the resident population

The number of children below school age remains fairly stable. The population of school-age children is now increasing slowly. The younger working population aged 16-29 years is falling, whereas the older working population (aged 30-59 years for women and 30-64 years for men) is increasing. The most elderly group of pensioners (aged 85 years and over) continues to increase and represents a growing proportion of all pensioners.

Fertility statistics - aspects of relevance for health care

Provisional data indicate that, in 1992, 785,000 conceptions occurred to women resident in England, a 3% fall from the actual figure in 1991, with an overall provisional conception rate of 76.4 per 1,000 women aged 15-44 years. In 1994, there were 628,956 live births in England - 1% fewer than in 1993, and the fourth successive year to show a fall. Based on provisional data, 149,640 abortions were performed in 1994 on women resident in England, a fall of 1% compared with 1993.

Mortality

Deaths registered in England increased from 522,656 in 1992 to 540,554 in 1993, a rise of 3.4%, and then fell by 4.5% to 516,095 in 1994. For most age-groups, mortality rates fell during the 1980s in males and females, but an 8% increase was seen for men aged 15-44 years between 1985 and 1990; since 1990, the mortality rate among men in this age-group has fallen by 9%.

Prevalence of disease in the community

In 1991-92, the overall consulting rate in general practice was 86% for women and 70% for men[16]. Consulting rates for all malignant disease rose from 68 to 90 per 10,000 between 1981-82 and 1991-92. For circulatory diseases, consulting rates rose from 850 to 931 per 10,000 over the same period, although new incidence of uncomplicated hypertension, cerebrovascular disease, and acute myocardial infarction fell. Despite an overall reduction in consulting rates for mental disorders, consulting rates for serious mental disorders increased from 72 to 113 per 10,000.

In 1993, 34% of respondents to the General Household Survey (GHS)[17] reported a long-standing illness, 20% a limiting long-standing illness, and 14% restricted activity during the two weeks before interview. The proportion of the population with a limiting long-term illness may vary between different ethnic groups and geographical area, according to data from the 1991 Census.

Infant and perinatal mortality

Provisional statistics for 1994 in England indicate that 3,842 babies died before the age of one year. The infant mortality rate was 6.1 per 1,000 live-births, the lowest ever recorded and a 3% fall from 1993. There were 3,583 stillbirths in 1994 compared with 3,621 in 1993; the stillbirth rate remained steady at 5.7 per 1,000 total births.

Trends in cancer incidence and mortality

Data from the 1988[18] and 1989[19] GHSs show that 1% of adults reported cancer as a cause for long-standing illness, and a similar figure is indicated by the Office of Population Censuses and Surveys (OPCS) Longitudinal Study. There was an increase in incidence for all malignant neoplasms combined (excluding non-melanoma skin cancer) between 1979 and 1990. Registrations of malignant melanoma of the skin rose considerably for men and women over this period. When adjusted for age, lung cancer registration fell for males but increased for females between 1979 and 1990.

Trends in reporting congenital malformations

According to provisional data for 1994, the rate for malformed live births fell to 69.2 per 10,000 live-births, 17% lower than in 1993 and 39% lower than in 1990.

THE NATION'S HEALTH

Public health in England

The national Public Health Network continued to draw together public health skills and specialist knowledge to advance the public health. A new electronic communications system was set up to enable rapid communication between DH and providers of health care[20].

Regional perspective

Considerable activity to reorganise health authorities in England should ensure further emphasis on a public health function.

Inter-Departmental Group on Public Health

The Inter-Departmental Group on Public Health, chaired by the Chief Medical Officer, facilitates discussion and exchange of information on health issues across a wide range of Government Departments.

Urban and rural differences in health

A number of factors associated with city life can contribute to poor health, but people living in rural areas may also have particular needs[16,21].

Variations in health

Variations in health may be seen in relation to geographical area, social class, ethnicity, occupation and gender. A better understanding of the underlying reasons for these variations is needed to enhance the health of the population as a whole.

Substance misuse

Progress towards the Health of the Nation targets[1] in smoking is in the right direction, with the exception of smoking and young people, where results are disappointing. Some 12% of young people aged 11-15 years were regular cigarette smokers in 1994[22]. A three-year national anti-smoking campaign launched in December focuses on the role of parents in encouraging young people not to take up the smoking habit[23]. Alcohol consumption and drinking behaviour seem to have changed little in recent years, but among current drinkers 9% of men and 5% of women are classified as problem drinkers[24,25]. A Task Force to review services for drug misusers was established in April, and a Green Paper, *Tackling Drugs Together*[15], was published in October.

Nutrition

The Committee on Medical Aspects of Food Policy published reports on *Weaning and the weaning diet*[26] and on *Nutritional aspects of cardiovascular disease*[27]. The Nutrition Task Force published several documents to help to achieve Health of the Nation nutrition targets[28,29,30,31]. A nutrition survey of people aged 65 years and over, and a survey of infant feeding in Asians, were started. The Nutrition Programme Committee held a meeting of experts to develop future priorities for the programme.

Health of people in later life

DH continues to promote work on sickness and disability prevention among elderly people.

Health of black and ethnic minorities

The NHS Ethnic Health Unit provided £1 million to fund innovative projects during 1994, with particular emphasis on improving communication between local ethnic groups and health authorities. Progress continued in research and monitoring, and the NHS Executive continued to implement its programme of action for ethnic minority NHS staff.

Health of men

Two themes in the Health of the Nation[1] - health alliances and healthy settings - are particularly relevant to target men effectively on health matters. An alliance of health and leisure organisations and the media should help to encourage physical activity and healthier lifestyles, and health promotion initiatives in the workplace offer the opportunity to promote healthier lifestyles in an appropriate setting for many men. A sub-group of the Chief Medical Officer's Health of the Nation Working Group has been established to look at variations in health in the five key areas of the health strategy and to identify action that DH and the NHS can take; gender variations are one of the areas being considered.

Health of adolescents

Following the special chapter in last year's Report[6], various initiatives to promote adolescent health are under way or planned, including a conference on the 'Health of the Young Nation'. Services for young people and adolescent risk behaviour are among DH's research priorities.

THE STRATEGY FOR HEALTH

Introduction

The Health of the Nation strategy[1] emphasises the benefits and importance of preventing ill-health, as well as treating it, and sets targets for health gain in five key areas. Most of these targets are timed for the year 2000, and in most areas data monitoring indicates steady progress towards meeting them.

Key areas and targets

Coronary heart disease and stroke: Risk factors for coronary heart disease (CHD) and stroke were again analysed in the report of the 1992 Health Survey for England[32] and in epidemiological overviews[33,34]. Ways to encourage physical activity are being explored.

Cancers: The NHS breast screening programme underpins the strategy of reducing breast cancer mortality and all screening centres have completed the first round of screening with a higher number of cancers detected by the programme than expected. Coverage of the cervical screening programme is now high[35], and a national co-ordinator has been appointed to develop quality assurance. Activity to support the skin cancer target included a campaign by the Health Education Authority (HEA) to promote improved awareness of the dangers of over-exposure to sunlight. Lung cancer is the most common form of cancer in men and the third most common form in women[36]; at least 80% of cases are associated with cigarette smoking.

Mental illness: The first in a series of reports on the National Psychiatric Morbidity Survey, showing prevalence rates of psychiatric disorders, was published[37]. Progress was made towards more effective implementation of mental health policy, and there was an encouraging reduction in suicide rates.

HIV/AIDS and sexual health: Work continues to sustain progress towards targets and to improve monitoring of equipment sharing among drug misusers.

Accidents: Encouraging progress has been made towards mortality reduction targets among children and young people, but deaths from accidents among elderly people appeared to rise; further investigation into these figures is under way.

Implementation

Priorities for the NHS: The strategy for health continues to be a top priority for the NHS within its *Priorities and Planning Guidance*[38,39], and Regional Health Authorities have agreed local targets to contribute towards the national targets as well as reflecting additional local health priorities.

Local health alliances: Health alliances are encouraged and identified through regional and national aspects of the Health Alliances Award Scheme. Judging for the first year of the scheme will take place in early 1995.

Healthy settings: Various healthy settings where health promotion activity might profitably be focused are receiving attention from relevant Government Departments in conjunction with DH.

Inter-Departmental co-operation: The strategy continues to be taken forward across Government Departments with a special Cabinet sub-committee to co-ordinate its implementation, monitoring and development.

The way ahead

For the immediate future, work will focus on those areas where monitoring shows that concentrated effort is needed and on further development of a communications strategy to promote and to co-ordinate the initiative, with selection of a succession of themes where work can focus; the first of these is to be the health of the young nation.

HEALTH IN THE WORKPLACE

Introduction

In the past, particularly following the Industrial Revolution, working conditions in Britain were often poor and health suffered as a result. Political will and economic progress have led to a well-developed regulatory system for health and safety at work, and enormous strides have been made in the prevention of serious and disabling disease and injury. Nevertheless, changing patterns of work-related illness present new challenges, and despite many advances there is still an appreciable national burden of ill-health and injury from work-related activities[40,41].

Occupational health today

The changing industrial base and pattern of employment: The structure of employment is changing, with a decline in heavy manufacturing and a rise in service sector employment; part-time and self-employment have increased, females now represent 44% of the labour force compared with 38% twenty years ago, and small businesses now account for over 30% of total employment.

Societal changes and public expectations: Workers have a right to a safe and healthy working environment. However, the perception and acceptance of risks by individuals and society depend on several factors and may vary over time.

International influences: An EC Framework Directive giving employers a number of new general duties with an impact on occupational health was implemented in the UK by the Management of Health and Safety at Work Regulations 1992[42]. The World Health Organization's (WHO's) policy for Europe includes reference to the health of people at work[43].

What is occupational health?

The effect of work on health: Almost half the population is employed and work is an important factor in people's health. Causes of illness in the workplace can be hard to identify, but the key to prevention lies in a thorough and well-informed assessment of risks, implementation of control measures and early identification of problems through health surveillance.

The effect of health on work: Health assessments of fitness for work are designed to ensure that individuals are physically and mentally fit to perform tasks effectively and without risk to themselves or colleagues.

Health promotion: With about half the population working, many of whom spend about half their waking hours at work on working days, there is an opportunity at places of employment to encourage healthier lifestyle choices.

Legislative and organisational framework

The Health and Safety at Work Act etc. 1974 places general duties on all people at work. Employers must ensure, so far as is reasonably practicable, the health, safety and welfare at work of their employees and others who may be affected by their activities. Employees have a duty to take reasonable care for their own safety and that of others. Employers must also follow general duties laid down in the Management of Health and Safety at Work Regulations 1992[42]. The Health and Safety Commission (HSC) and the Health and Safety Executive (HSE) promote, oversee and enforce these laws.

Information about occupational ill-health

No single source of information about occupational illness can provide the full statistical picture. The five main sources are the Industrial Injuries Scheme, voluntary reporting by the medical profession, the Labour Force Surveys conducted by OPCS, national mortality data and the statutory system introduced by the Reporting of Injuries, Diseases and Dangerous Occurrences Regulations (RIDDOR) 1986[44].

Main occupational health hazards, diseases and disorders

Chemical risks and diseases: Some classic occupational diseases such as byssinosis (from cotton dust) have fallen to very low levels. Pneumoconiosis is also falling, but more slowly - perhaps because of a long latency between exposure and onset of disease. Deaths attributed to asbestos exposure have been rising, but again a long latency period may reflect past industrial conditions. Some other chemical carcinogens have been associated with specific industries or jobs. Occupational asthma and dermatitis are now the major causes of ill-health as a result of current exposures to chemicals in the workplace. Acute poisoning by industrial chemicals is still a risk.

Physical risks and diseases: Musculo-skeletal disorders form the largest single category of work-related illnesses in Britain by a wide margin, with an estimated annual prevalence of 880,000 causing 5.5 million working days to be lost each year[40]. Work-related upper limb disorders and back injuries caused by manual handling are particular challenges. Hand-arm vibration may lead to vibration white finger or a more extensive syndrome; the effects of whole-body vibration are unclear. Noise exposure can lead to noise-induced hearing loss and tinnitus. Exposure to ionising radiation can occur in a wide range of occupations. The effects of non-ionising radiation, including ultraviolet (UV) and visible light, infra-red, microwave, radiofrequency and laser beams, and electromagnetic fields, are being researched. Extremes of heat and cold, and work with compressed air, may affect some workers.

Biological hazards and diseases: Micro-organisms may cause disease directly or have allergic and toxic effects. Blood-borne infections are a potential hazard to workers at risk of exposure to blood, body fluids or blood-contaminated sharp objects. Classic occupational zoonoses such as anthrax and brucellosis are now rare, but zoonoses such as cryptosporidiosis may affect 8,000 people each year (although the proportion due to occupational exposure is unclear). DH has assessors on the Advisory Committee on Genetic Modification and the Advisory Committee on Releases to the Environment.

Work-related psychosocial risks and ill-health: Studies of minor psychiatric morbidity in working populations indicate a prevalence of 270-370 per 1,000 employees[45], which may be higher during periods of occupational instability[46]; it is a major determinant of sickness absence. Certain characteristics of jobs and the working environment may be stressful and potentially harmful to health[47], but other factors within the workplace may act as sources of support. As part of the Health of the Nation strategy[1], DH has worked to increase employers' awareness of these issues, and produced *A guide to mental health in the workplace*[48] and *ABC of mental health in the workplace*[49].

Rural issues: Although the countryside may not generally be considered a workplace, agricultural workers and others may be exposed to a wide range of occupational health and safety risks.

Effects of health on work

Some jobs have specific criteria for medical standards of fitness to help to ensure that employees carry out tasks safely without undue harm to themselves or others. However, for most types of work there are no clearly defined criteria for fitness on medical grounds and interpretations may vary. A proper assessment of the working environment and duties involved, and a health assessment appropriate to the work to be done, should ensure no unnecessary restrictions being placed on employability[50,51].

Health promotion

The workplace is a useful population for health promotion activity and local alliances to this end are being strengthened by the Health of the Nation initiative[1].

Occupational health services

Occupational health services (OHSs) offer a specialist advisory service to promote health and safety for management and employees alike. Greater emphasis is now placed on advisory rather than treatment services; giving advice on prevention as well as protection; health surveillance; and multi-disciplinary expertise.

Ethics and confidentiality

The impartiality, integrity and confidentiality of OHSs must be recognised and maintained[52].

Health of NHS staff

A healthy workforce is essential for the NHS to provide high-quality health care and improve the health of the population. The Health at Work in the NHS (HAWNHS) initiative was launched in 1992 to pursue Health of the Nation targets[1] in NHS workplaces, and to encourage moves towards those targets outside the NHS.

Responsibilities and training

OHSs have independent professional status and should report to senior management; they need staff with appropriate specialist qualifications, depending on the type of service that needs to be provided.

Audit in occupational health

Audit of the structure, process or outcome of practice assists the development of improved clinical standards and guidelines, contributes to continuing professional development and helps to meet the needs of the client as user of the service.

Research

The HSE's occupational health research programme is informed by the priority areas and objectives identified by the HSC's Health Risk Reviews. The British Occupational Health Research Foundation is setting up a series of workshops to identify and discuss long-term challenges.

Future developments and emerging issues

Strategic health risk reviews: A major review of ten principal occupational health risks by the HSC and the HSE identified strategic priorities and set out proposals for action on each health risk.

Reproductive health: The HSE has established a research programme to investigate whether exposure to chemicals is affecting male fertility.

Genetic screening: Certain inherited traits may increase the risk of acquiring occupational disease, and ability to identify such traits is likely to increase rapidly. However, other uses could be made of genetic screening and the topic raises important legal and ethical issues which have not yet been resolved.

Environmental issues: In March, the Faculties of Occupational Medicine and Public Health Medicine of the Royal College of Physicians of London set up a joint Standing Group on the Environment. The UK is drafting a national action plan in response to the WHO's Environmental Health Action Plan for Europe.

International issues: Recent European initiatives in occupational health include a European Association for Schools of Occupational Medicine. A European network of occupational health nursing educators and teachers holds meetings and workshops, and other international scientific and research conferences are planned.

The way ahead: Much of the burden of work-related ill-health is preventable and a greater appreciation of possible risks, and a better understanding of how to manage them effectively, will benefit employers and employees alike. The rapid development and implementation of new technological advances in industry brings with it new challenges for doctors and other health care professionals.

HEALTH CARE

Needs, effectiveness and outcomes

Health needs assessment: The assessment of health needs continues to develop, with publication of a series of epidemiologically based needs reviews[53]

Basic sources of information: A number of major surveys have been initiated, completed or published during 1994. Taken together, data from these surveys - which cover topics such as cardiovascular disease and its risk factors[32], psychiatric morbidity[37] and diet and nutrition[27] - provide a valuable picture of the underlying health of the general population.

National confidential enquiries: The Reports for 1992[54] and 1993[55] described the purposes of confidential enquiry, summarised the principles of the methods used, and outlined the progress of the five national confidential enquiries. Progress was maintained during 1994 . The report of the Confidential Enquiries into Maternal Deaths in the United Kingdom[56] was published in January.

Quality of service and effectiveness of care: The transfer of good research evidence into changed and improved health service practice is a key goal. The role of clinical audit continues to be developed.

National Casemix Office and NHS Centre for Coding and Classification: The National Casemix Office and the NHS Centre for Coding and Classification continue to refine and to promulgate coding systems within the NHS.

Clinical outcomes: The population health outcome indicators[57] have been updated and will be published with the Public Health Common Data Set in 1995. Their use will be evaluated over the subsequent year. Work has started to develop 'ideal' outcome indicators for 10 health topics, along with a composite indicator and a set of clinical quality indicators.

Primary health care

Organisation of primary care: Considerable progress has been made to focus primary care services on health promotion and to establish electronic links between practices and Family Health Services Authorities (FHSAs). Practices are working more closely together to strengthen local services for patients, and steady recruitment of GP practices to the fundholding scheme continues.

Prescribing: Improvements in quality and cost-effectiveness have been seen in some areas of prescribing. Nevertheless, the near 10% real-terms increase of the primary care drugs bill in 1993/94 emphasises the importance of rational prescribing[58].

Professional development: Clinical audit and continuing professional development are closely linked; a report of the primary health care working group of the Clinical Outcomes Group is expected next year.

The way ahead: As the purchasing of secondary care and community services becomes increasingly led by general practitioners (GPs), a major challenge will be to secure the continued provision of good quality services within primary care itself.

Hospital services

Specialised services: A review of the central purchase of highly specialised services advised a continued need for Supra-Regional Services arrangements and made recommendations about central purchasing of other specialised services; consultation on these recommendations is under way.

Cancer: The Chief Medical Officer's Expert Advisory Group published a consultation document on the commissioning of cancer services, which is being considered by Ministers.

Thromboprophylaxis: A conference on thromboprophylaxis was held at the Royal College of Surgeons of England in June, and the subject has been recognised as a priority for further research.

Minimal access surgery: A report issued by the Scottish Office Home and Health Department made recommendations about clinical and management aspects of laparoscopic general surgery. The Standing Medical Advisory Committee (SMAC) is considering the report with a view to providing further advice about minimal access surgery.

Osteoporosis: The Advisory Group on Osteoporosis prepared a report; following consultation, this should be published early in 1995.

Transplantation: The NHS Organ Donor Register was launched in October. In December, a pilot scheme was set up in GP practices in two FHSAs to enable patients registering with a GP to record their donor wishes.

Diabetes mellitus

The Clinical Standards Advisory Group reported on standards of clinical care for people with diabetes mellitus[59]. The joint DH/British Diabetic Association Task Force for diabetes mellitus made its second report in November.

Asthma

In October, Ministers announced a conference to be held in 1995 to improve the understanding of asthma. The 'Breathe Freely' campaign aims to reduce levels of occupational asthma.

Complementary medicine

The Chiropractors Act 1994[60] provides for the establishment of a General Chiropractic Council to develop, promote and regulate the profession of chiropractic.

Mental health

Mental health and primary care: A joint venture between DH, the Royal College of General Practitioners and the Gatsby Charitable Foundation has set up a national network of regional GP mental health fellows to advise primary care teams.

Occupational mental health: DH continued to emphasise the need for action on workplace mental health and published a resource pack for employers[49].

Confidential Inquiry into Homicides and Suicides: The Confidential Inquiry reported on 22 cases of homicide by people currently or previously under the care of the specialist psychiatric service[61].

Services for people with severe mental illness: A practical framework to establish the range of care needed to assess and to meet the needs of people with severe mental illness was prepared for the second edition of the Health of the Nation key area handbook on mental illness[62]. The Mental Health Task Force London project reviewed services in twelve London health districts, and the particular needs of people from different ethnic and cultural groups were emphasised.

Services for mentally disordered offenders: Expert Working Groups reported on high security psychiatric services[63] and on psychopathic disorder[64]. Increased numbers of mentally disordered people continue to transfer to health care from prisons under provisions of the Mental Health Act 1983[65]. More secure beds were provided, but pressures on availability have continued.

Mental health legislation: In October, DH issued a consultation paper to seek views on promoting the use of guardianship under the Mental Health Act 1983[65] or extending its powers. Following widespread consultation on supervised discharge, a Mental Health Bill was announced in the Queen's Speech in November.

Maternity and child health services

Implementation of 'Changing Childbirth': Following the Government decision to implement the recommendations of the Report of the Expert Maternity Group [66], DH appointed an implementation team and established an Advisory Group. Work also began on ways to measure whether the indicators of change listed in the report were reached.

Confidential Enquiries into Maternal Deaths: The *Report on Confidential Enquiries into Maternal Deaths in the United Kingdom 1988-1990* was published in January[56].

Folic acid and the prevention of neural tube defects: Licensed 400 microgram folic acid supplements became available, and may now be advertised for prevention of neural tube defects.

Human Fertilisation and Embryology Authority: The regulatory work of the Authority was conducted effectively[67], with public consultation on the use of donated ovarian tissue in embryo research and assisted conception[68].

Sudden infant death syndrome: After renewed allegations that toxic gases could be generated by microbial action upon cot mattresses and cause sudden infant death, the Chief Medical Officer set up an expert group to review the evidence[69].

Prophylaxis of vitamin K deficiency bleeding in infants: The Chief Medical Officer met representatives of medical and nursing professional bodies to discuss concerns over the administration of vitamin K. It was agreed that advice setting out good practice could best be prepared by the relevant professions and that it should take into account the results of research expected to be published in the near future.

Retinopathy of prematurity: The unfavourable outcome of retinopathy of prematurity can now be reduced significantly by treatment, and DH has commissioned a nationwide research, training and audit programme to improve the outcome for babies at high risk.

Paediatric intensive care: Research continues into the factors which influence the survival of critically ill children, and on the content and organisation of paediatric intensive care within the NHS[70].

Confidential Enquiry into Stillbirths and Deaths in Infancy: Good progress was maintained on the collection of data, the programme of confidential enquiries and the study into sudden unexpected deaths in infancy. The National Advisory Body began preparing its report for 1993, due to be published early in 1995.

Congenital malformations: Sporadic reports of apparently unusual occurrences of a number of congenital anomalies raised public and Parliamentary concerns, and much speculation on possible causes. The Department has commissioned studies into anophthalmia and limb reduction defects.

Gene Therapy Advisory Committee: The Gene Therapy Advisory Committee met five times in 1994. Ten protocols for gene therapy had been approved by December.

Code of Practice on special educational needs and circulars on 'Pupils with problems': The Department for Education and the Department of Health published a number of guidance documents on the identification and assessment of special educational needs[71], and a set of circulars on 'Pupils with problems' [72,73,74].

Learning disabilities

A booklet to enable the implementation of the Health of the Nation policy[1] for people with learning disabilities was prepared and will be published during 1995.

Disability and rehabilitation

Developments included National Continence Week; a publication on pressure sores[75]; a report on the Department's brain injury rehabilitation initiative[76]; the establishment of research projects to develop targets; and discussion on the devolution to the NHS of the DH budget for the supply of environmental control systems. Local purchasers of health services were asked to improve services for people with physical disabilities.

Prison health care

The devolution of responsibility for the effective delivery of health care to local prison managers has encouraged even closer working with the NHS, although the Directorate of Health Care for Prisoners retains its policy role and has taken on responsibility for health and safety within the Prison Service. The Prison Service drugs strategy was launched and additional health care standards issued.

London Implementation Group

Improvements to family doctor and community health services continued to be made in London. Nearly 1,000 such schemes are now planned or under way in the London Initiative Zone.

COMMUNICABLE DISEASES

HIV infection and AIDS

Data reported for HIV infection and AIDS showed a similar pattern to previous years. In 1994, further data from the unlinked anonymous HIV surveys from 1990 to 1993 became available and showed a significant rise in prevalence among pregnant women; whilst prevalence is highest in London, HIV-1 infection is present in high-risk groups in every region surveyed. In March, DH published revised guidance on management of HIV-infected health care workers[77]. Guidance on antenatal voluntary named HIV testing was published in June[78].

Other sexually transmitted diseases

The total number of new cases seen at genito-urinary medicine clinics continues to rise, although the proportion actually diagnosed as having a sexually transmitted disease (STD) fell in 1993, and the number of reports of many STDs decreased. A fall in the total reports of gonorrhoea by just under 24% in 1992 resulted in a rate below the target of 49 per 100,000 population aged 15-64 years set by the Health of the Nation strategy[1]; a further fall of 17% during 1993 reduced this rate to 38 per 100,000. There was a rise in reports of first attacks of herpes simplex and of reports of recurrent attacks, particularly among women.

Immunisation

In November, a nationwide mass measles/rubella immunisation campaign was carried out. On the basis of UK epidemiological data and the experience of other countries, it was considered highly probable that there would be a measles epidemic in early 1995. Because the age-group at highest risk was school-aged children, the immunisation campaign was targeted at children aged 5 to 16 years, and was delivered through school health services. Measles/rubella vaccine was used to prevent the measles epidemic and to bring forward the elimination of rubella by approximately 5 years. The target population for England was 7.17 million children: immunisation coverage of 92% was achieved and the impact on measles has been dramatic.

Viral hepatitis

Viral hepatitis is a notifiable disease. In 1994 a provisional total of 3,734 cases were reported to the OPCS from England, a fall of 33% compared with the previous year. Of these, 2,726 were due to hepatitis A and 532 due to hepatitis B.

Influenza

Influenza activity remained at low levels throughout the year. A sharp increase in acute respiratory infections in December was mainly due to respiratory syncytial virus and *Mycoplasma pneumoniae*.

Tuberculosis

A new national survey of tuberculosis notifications revealed that notification rates in the white population and in those of Indian subcontinent origin have continued to decline, although the total number of cases in the latter increased. The notification rate in those of 'other' ethnic origin has increased since 1988.

Plague

In October, DH responded to reports of outbreaks of plague in India by immediate strengthening of port health controls and heightened surveillance of suspected cases. No case was identified in this country.

Necrotising fasciitis

Following a cluster of cases of necrotising fasciitis, enhanced surveillance of invasive group A streptococcal infection was begun to allay public concern.

Antibiotic resistance and hospital-acquired infection

Guidance on the management of infections by methicillin-resistant *Staphylococcus aureus*[79] has been endorsed[80] and guidance on *Clostridium difficile* infections was published in September[81].

Foodborne and waterborne diseases

Notifications of food poisoning to the OPCS rose by 18% between 1993 and 1994. The number of laboratory isolations of *Campylobacter* rose by 13%, but isolations of *Salmonella*, verocytotoxin-producing *Escherichia coli* (VTEC) 0157, and *Listeria* remained at much the same level as in 1993. *Salmonella typhimurium* DT104 became the second most common *Salmonella*, and investigations began into the reasons for the rise in human illness associated with this organism. The Advisory Committee on the Microbiological Safety of Food completed its report on the significance of VTEC as a foodborne pathogen[12]. The microbiological quality of drinking water remains high with few outbreaks of disease attributable to public water supplies.

Travel-related disease

1,887 cases of malaria were imported into the UK, nearly two-thirds due to the more severe falciparum malaria. Reported imported illness also included 281 cases of hepatitis A, 201 cases of typhoid, 17 cases of cholera and a variety of other tropical diseases.

ENVIRONMENTAL HEALTH AND TOXICOLOGY

Chemical and physical agents in the environment

Small Area Health Statistics Unit: In 1994, the Small Area Health Statistics Unit completed an investigation of the incidence of cancer and mortality near the petrochemical works at Baglan Bay, South Wales, and a study of cancer incidence near all municipal incinerators in Great Britain. Further advances in the methodology for investigating health statistics in small areas have also been made.

Air pollution: Sufficient epidemiological evidence has arisen to give cause for concern about the possible health effects of current levels of airborne particles. During 1994, the Department of the Environment's Expert Panel on Air Quality Standards has recommended standards for benzene, 1,3-butadiene, ozone and carbon monoxide. A recommendation on airborne particles is expected during 1995.

Institute for Environment and Health: The Institute for Environment and Health held several workshops and produced two reports on air pollution and health during the year[82,83].

Committee on Medical Aspects of Radiation in the Environment: The Committee issued a statement about the raised incidence of certain childhood cancers near Dounreay, Scotland[84].

Environment and health: DH participated in the Second Ministerial Conference on Environment and Health in Helsinki, and the International Conference on Chemical Safety in Stockholm.

Surveillance of diseases possibly due to non-infectious environmental hazards: DH is considering recommendations of a Working Group set up to consider whether, and if so which, diseases might be appropriate for surveillance of non-infectious environmental hazards.

Toxicological safety

Food chemical hazards: New guidelines on the management of outbreaks of foodborne illness were published[85].

Food carcinogen prioritisation: A scheme to establish priorities for action among chemical carcinogens in food was agreed.

Peanut anaphylaxis: DH liaises with the Ministry of Agriculture, Fisheries and Food to ensure that voluntary labelling of food packaging specifies all types of nut, to allow consumers to exercise choice when purchasing food.

Traditional remedies: DH drew clinicians' attention to the possibility that their patients may be taking traditional remedies in addition to allopathic medicines[86].

The Advisory Committee on Novel Foods and Processes: DH continues to provide support for medical, toxicological and nutritional aspects of the work of the Advisory Committee on Novel Foods and Processes (ACNFP).

Genetically modified food plants: During 1994, the ACNFP recommended food safety clearance of food products derived from genetically modified tomatoes, oilseed rape and soya.

Fat replacers: The ACNFP considered the assessment of novel fats for possible thrombotic effects.

Man-made mineral fibres: Carcinogenicity data on man-made mineral fibres used in domestic insulation were reviewed. Additional epidemiological data should become available in 1995.

Organization for Economic Co-operation and Development guidelines for testing chemicals for toxicity: These guidelines play a key role in the international harmonisation of methods to investigate chemical toxicity. Progress was made in genetic toxicology and in other areas.

Pesticides: The results of surveillance monitoring of foods for pesticide residues showed relatively few breaches of statutory limits[87,88,89]. Approvals for the use of lindane were examined during the year.

Veterinary drugs: Reports of adverse reactions to organophosphate sheep dips led to the introduction of a certificate of competence for sheep dippers to improve work practices. Tenders for appropriate research work have been invited.

MEDICAL EDUCATION, TRAINING AND STAFFING

Junior doctors' hours

During 1994, DH made considerable progress towards the elimination of hard-pressed on-call posts where junior doctors were contracted to work for over 72 hours per week. By the end of December there were only 1,793 such posts - a 72.5% fall in the nine months since 31 March.

'Achieving a Balance' and the Advisory Group on Medical and Dental Education, Training and Staffing

'Achieving a Balance' policy[90], together with the *'New Deal'*[91] and progress on implementation of *Hospital doctors: training for the future*[92] will now be considered with the advice of a new committee, the Advisory Group on Medical and Dental Education, Training and Staffing (AGMETS), set up during 1994.

Medical Manpower Standing Advisory Committee

The second report of the Committee is expected to be published in Summer 1995.

Equal opportunities for doctors

Current initiatives are likely to make training for hospital practice more attractive to young doctors who have family commitments. In December, flexible training schemes included 370 career registrars and 445 senior registrars.

Part-time consultants scheme

A second tranche of 85 new, centrally funded posts were approved under a scheme to promote part-time opportunities at consultant level[93].

New career structure for doctors in child health

New career structure guidance for a combined child health service was issued in March[94].

Postgraduate, continuing and specialist medical education

Work continued towards implementation of the report of the Working Party on Specialist Medical Training[92]. A Working Party considered principles for the operation of the new unified training grade, and other groups considered the report's implications for general practice, overseas doctors and academic and research medicine. A national conference was held to launch a consultative document on continuing medical and dental education.

Medical (Professional Performance) Bill

In November, the Government announced its intention[95] to introduce a Bill to amend the Medical Act 1983[96] to enable the General Medical Council to take action where a doctor's professional performance was seriously deficient for reasons not already covered by existing procedures[97].

Undergraduate medical and dental education

Special funding to help medical schools to implement changes in undergraduate medical education curricula has continued and was extended. Arrangements were made to review the Service Increment for Teaching and Research (SIFTR).

Doctors' performance

A Review Group, chaired by the Chief Medical Officer, has been considering the guidance and procedures relating to doctors whose performance appears to fall below acceptable standards.

Locum doctors

The Working Group on Hospital Locum Doctors reported in the autumn; its report will be published for consultation in 1995.

OTHER TOPICS OF INTEREST IN 1994

Medicines Control Agency

Role and performance: The role of the Medicines Control Agency (MCA) is to protect public health by ensuring that all medicines for human use meet stringent criteria of safety, quality and efficacy. The MCA met most of its targets and is among the fastest pharmaceutical licensing authorities in the world.

Control of UK clinical trials: Patients in clinical trials are protected by a system of authorisations and monitoring procedures; this system is under review.

Legal reclassification of medicinal products: In 1994, new arrangements were introduced to publish an amendment to the Prescription Only Medicine (POM) Order[98] twice a year. A number of medicines were released from prescription control.

Pharmaceutical developments in the European Community: The MCA maintained a leading role in EC licensing and implemented, on time, legislation setting up the new EC licensing system.

European Medicines Evaluation Agency

Preparatory work was undertaken for the new licensing system for medicines in the EC, which comes into force from 1 January 1995. The establishment in London of the European Medicines Evaluation Agency (EMEA) will support the new system.

Medical Devices Agency

The Medical Devices Agency (MDA) became an Executive Agency of DH in September. The MDA maintained a leading role in implementation of relevant EC legislation.

National Blood Authority

The National Blood Authority (NBA) took over management responsibility for the regional blood transfusion centres in England on 1 April. The NBA is now in the process of a proposed reorganisation of the transfusion centre network aimed at improving quality and the service provided.

National Biological Standards Board

The National Biological Standards Board (NBSB) has a statutory duty to maintain high standards of quality and reliability of biological substances used in medicine, to develop biological standards for such substances and to conduct associated research and development. The NBSB does this through its management of the National Institute for Biological Standards and Control (NIBSC). Work during the year included support of the influenza and measles/rubella immunisation campaigns, and the NIBSC was the first of the eight EC-designated European Control Testing Laboratories to achieve international accreditation to quality standard EN45001.

National Radiological Protection Board

The National Radiological Protection Board (NRPB) was set up to advance the acquisition of knowledge about the protection of mankind from radiation hazards (for both ionising and non-ionising radiation), and to provide information and advice in relation to protection from radiation hazards. During 1994, the NRPB worked to support the Health of the Nation initiative on skin cancer, and has issued specialist and public advice on various aspects of radiation. A new medical division was set up in October.

United Kingdom Transplant Support Service Authority

The UK Transplant Support Service Authority (UKTSSA) was established in 1994 to facilitate the matching and allocation of organs for transplantation.

Microbiological Research Authority

The Microbiological Research Authority, set up on 1 April, is a Special Health Authority which administers the Centre for Applied Microbiology and Research, Porton Down.

Creutzfeldt-Jakob Disease Surveillance Unit

The Creutzfeldt-Jakob Disease Surveillance Unit was established in 1990 in Edinburgh, and continues to monitor any changes in the incidence of Creutzfeldt-Jakob disease in human beings.

Bioethics

Local Research Ethics Committees: DH launched a standards initiative for Local Research Ethics Committees[99]. A consultative group examined ethical approval of multi-centre studies.

Bioethics in Europe: The Council of Europe draft Bioethics Convention was issued for consultation in July.

Genetic screening: The House of Commons Select Committee on Science and Technology began its Inquiry into Human Genetics; this Inquiry will encompass genetic screening.

Draft guidance on confidentiality: DH issued for wide consultation draft guidance on the confidentiality, use and disclosure of personal health information. The responses are being analysed with a view to issuing definitive guidance during 1995.

House of Lords Select Committee on Medical Ethics: The Committee considered issues surrounding the end of life, recommending no change to the law on euthanasia[100]; the Government supported the Committee's view[101].

Research and development

White Paper on Science, Engineering and Technology: The development of the Department's research and development (R&D) strategy continues to be informed by the implementation of the White Paper *Realising Our Potential* [102,103].

***Research for health*:** DH's centrally Commissioned Programme now focuses on a range of strategic issues with future programmes of work now in planning.

***Developments in the NHS research and development programme*:** NHS R&D will take account of new organisational structures[104,105] and a radical new 'single stream' funding mechanism for R&D will be introduced. Research results continue to be disseminated effectively.

Dental health

Dental health of the nation: An oral health strategy for England[106] was published alongside the Green Paper *Improving NHS Dentistry*[107]; it emphasises the need for early detection and prevention of oral diseases, and quality of care.

General dental services: The Green Paper *Improving NHS Dentistry*[107] sets out proposals for reform of the dental remuneration system. A consultation period ended in November and the Government is now considering the result.

Community dental services: The provision of community dental services is now firmly established within NHS Trusts.

Hospital dental services: The number of hospital dentists in England rose by 2.6% between September 1992 and September 1993. New outpatient referrals to consultant clinics fell by 1.1% in 1993/94 compared with 1992/93.

Continuing education and training for dentists: On 1 October, there were 513 trainees in 47 regionally based vocational training schemes.

Dental research: Dental research commissioned by DH included a study of diet and oral health among people aged 65 years and over, and a follow-up[108] to the 1988 Adult Dental Health Survey[109] to investigate the longevity of dental crowns.

INTERNATIONAL HEALTH

England, Europe and health

Many of the health challenges encountered in England and the rest of the UK are also found in the rest of Europe. The UK continues to co-operate in health matters with other countries in the EC and international organisations such as the WHO and the Council of Europe.

The European Community

The Council of Health Ministers: The Health Council considered European Commission proposals on extension of the 'Europe against Cancer' programme, and work on AIDS and other communicable diseases, drug dependence and health promotion.

EC/WHO/Council of Europe: Close co-operation between the EC, the WHO and the Council of Europe continued during 1994.

European Economic Area: The establishment of the European Economic Area (EEA) extended the Single European Market, including EC rules on professional qualifications, to Austria, Finland, Iceland, Norway and Sweden.

Free movement of people: EC Regulations to co-ordinate recognition of qualifications and the movement of patients continued to operate satisfactorily.

Channel Tunnel and port health checks: The Public Health (International Trains) Regulations[109,110] came into force to protect public health against the transmission of disease via the Channel Tunnel.

Draft Directive on Data Protection: Negotiations on this draft Directive continued during 1994 and helpful amendments relating to health data were agreed.

Smoking: Discussions continued on advertising, excise duty and other measures to reduce tobacco consumption.

Elderly and disabled people: During 1994, an evaluation programme on the 1993 'European Year of Older People and Solidarity Between Generations' was undertaken. UK participants played an active and enthusiastic part in HELIOS II, the third Community action programme for disabled people.

AIDS and HIV infection: Actions under the 'Europe Against AIDS' programme continued, and the programme was extended while future measures are debated.

Research and information technology: A new four-year EC research and technological development programme was agreed, containing as before a biomedical and health theme.

Food safety: Consultation began on UK Regulations implementing the EC General Food Hygiene Directive.

Medical Devices Directives: The UK continued to implement the provisions of the different Medical Devices Directives.

Relations with Central and Eastern Europe

The UK continued to foster links with Central and Eastern Europe and to offer assistance, often through Health Co-operation Agreements. In addition, Bulgaria, the Czech Republic, Hungary, Poland, Rumania and Slovakia, in preparation for ultimate European Union membership, were permitted to join in EC programmes, including those in public health.

Council of Europe

The UK continued to participate actively in the work of the Council of Europe Health Committee and its Bioethics Committee. Experts from the UK also contributed to the work of select committees and working groups covering a wide range of health issues. The Council of Europe Pompidou Group held its 10th Ministerial Conference and 2nd Pan-European Ministerial Conference in February.

Organization for Economic Co-operation and Development

The Organization for Economic Co-operation and Development (OECD) held a high-level conference on healthcare reform at which the Secretary of State for Health represented the UK.

The Commonwealth

The Chief Medical Officer led a delegation to the Commonwealth Health Ministers' meeting which preceded the World Health Assembly.

World Health Organization

European Regional Committee: Dr Jo Asvall was nominated as the European region's Regional Director for a third consecutive five-year term.

Executive Board: In January, the Board considered WHO's response to global change and the future of the Programme Committee. In May, members were appointed to two global change sub-committees; the Chief Medical Officer was elected to the Administration, Budget and Finance Committee.

World Health Assembly: In May, the World Health Assembly adopted the recommendations of the Executive Board's Working Group on WHO's response to global change. This Group, chaired by the Chief Medical Officer, had sought to develop a new strategic budget as a means of allowing greater transparency in the way in which the Organization conducted its operations at all levels.

References

1. Department of Health. *The Health of the Nation: a strategy for health in England.* London: HMSO, 1992 (Cm. 1986).
2. Department of Health. *On the State of the Public Health: the annual report of the Chief Medical Officer of the Department of Health for the year 1992.* London: HMSO, 1993; 2.

3. Department of Health. *On the State of the Public Health: the annual report of the Chief Medical Officer of the Department of Health for the year 1993*. London: HMSO, 1994; 2.

4. Department of Health. *On the State of the Public Health: the annual report of the Chief Medical Officer of the Department of Health for the year 1993*. London: HMSO, 1994; 6.

5. Expert Advisory Group on Cancer. *A policy framework for commissioning cancer services*. London: Department of Health, 1995.

6. Department of Health. *On the State of the Public Health: the annual report of the Chief Medical Officer of the Department of Health for the year 1993*. London: HMSO, 1994; 5, 74-112.

7. Department of Health. *Health of the Nation: what you can do about it*. Heywood (Lancashire): Department of Health, 1995.

8. General Medical Council. *Tomorrow's doctors: recommendations on undergraduate medical education*. London: General Medical Council, 1993.

9. Department of Health. *Hospital doctors: training for the future: the report of the working group on specialist medical training*. London: Department of Health, 1993. Chair: Dr Kenneth Calman.

10. Department of Health. *Hospital doctors: training for the future: supplementary reports on general practice, overseas doctors and academic and research medicine*. Heywood (Lancashire): Department of Health, 1995 (Executive Letter: EL(95)62).

11. NHS Executive. *High security psychiatric services: changes in funding and organisation*. Leeds: NHS Executive, 1995.

12. Advisory Committee on the Microbiological Safety of Food. *Report on verocytotoxin-producing Escherichia coli*. London: HMSO, 1995.

13. Department of Health. *Chief Medical Officer advises vulnerable groups to avoid raw milk*. London: Department of Health, 1995 (Press Release: H95/278).

14. NHS Health Advisory Service. *Together we stand: the commissioning, role and management of child and adolescent mental health services*. London: HMSO, 1995.

15. Lord President's Office. *Tackling Drugs Together: a consultation document on a strategy for England: 1995-1998*. London: HMSO, 1994 (Cm. 2678).

16. McCormick A, Fleming D, Charlton J. *Morbidity Statistics from General Practice: fourth national study: 1991-92*. London: HMSO (in press).

17. Office of Population Censuses and Surveys. *General Household Survey 1993*. London: HMSO (in press).

18. Office of Population Censuses and Surveys. *General Household Survey 1988*. London: HMSO, 1990 (Series GHS no. 19).

19. Office of Population Censuses and Surveys. *General Household Survey 1989*. London: HMSO, 1991 (Series GHS no. 20).

20. Department of Health. *Communications with the profession*. Heywood (Lancashire): Department of Health, 1994 (Professional Letter: PL/CMO(94)3).

21. Watt IS, Franks AJ, Sheldon TA. Health and health care of rural populations in the UK: is it better or worse? *J Epidemiol Commun Health* 1994; **48:** 16-21.

22. Office of Population Censuses and Surveys. *Smoking among secondary school children in England in 1994: an enquiry carried out by the Social Survey Division of OPCS on behalf of the Department of Health*. London: HMSO (in press).

23. Department of Health. *Smoke-free for health: an action plan to achieve the Health of the Nation targets on smoking*. Heywood (Lancashire): Department of Health, 1994.

24. Office of Population Censuses and Surveys. *Health Survey for England 1992*. London: HMSO, 1994.

25. Office of Population Censuses and Surveys. *General Household Survey 1992*. London: HMSO, 1994 (GHS no. 23).

26. Department of Health. *Weaning and the weaning diet: report of the Working Group on the Weaning Diet of the Committee on Medical Aspects of Food Policy*. London: HMSO, 1994. (Report on Health and Social Subjects no. 45.)

27. Department of Health. *Nutritional aspects of cardiovascular disease: report of the Cardiovascular Review Group*. London: HMSO, 1994. (Report on Health and Social Subjects no. 46.)

28. Department of Health. *Eat Well! An action plan from the Nutrition Task Force to achieve the Health of the Nation targets on diet and nutrition*. Heywood (Lancashire): Department of Health, 1994. Chair: Professor Dame Barbara Clayton.

29. Department of Health. *Nutrition and health: a management handbook for the NHS*. London: Department of Health, 1994.

30. Health Education Authority. *The National Food Guide: the balance of good health*. London: Health Education Authority, 1994.

31. Department of Health. *Nutrition: core curriculum for nutrition in the education of health professionals*. London: Department of Health, 1994.

32. Office of Population Censuses and Surveys. *Health Survey for England 1992*. London: HMSO, 1994.

33. Department of Health, Central Health Monitoring Unit. *Coronary heart disease: an epidemiological overview*. London: Department of Health, 1994.

34. Department of Health, Central Health Monitoring Unit. *Stroke: an epidemiological overview*. London: Department of Health, 1994.

35. Department of Health. *Cervical cytology 1993/94. Summary information from Form KC53, England*. London: Department of Health (in press).

36. Office of Population Censuses and Surveys. *Cancer statistics registrations: registrations of cancer diagnosed: England and Wales: 1989*. London: Department of Health, 1994 (Series MB1 no. 22).

37. Meltzer H. *The prevalence of psychiatric morbidity among adults aged 16-64 living in private households in Great Britain.* London: OPCS, 1994 (OPCS Surveys of Psychiatric Morbidity in Great Britain; Bulletin 1).
38. Department of Health. *Priorities and planning guidance 1994/95.* Leeds: NHS Management Executive, 1993 (Executive Letter: EL(93)54).
39. Department of Health. *Priorities and planning guidance 1995/96.* Leeds: NHS Executive, 1994 (Executive Letter: EL(94)55).
40. Office of Population Censuses and Surveys. *Labour Force Survey 1990.* London: HMSO, 1993.
41. Health and Safety Executive. *The costs to the British economy of work accidents and work-related ill health.* London: Health and Safety Executive, 1994.
42. *Management of Health and Safety at Work Regulations 1992.* London: HMSO, 1992.
43. World Health Organization. *'Health for all' targets: the health policy for Europe, updated edn.,* Copenhagen: WHO, 1994.
44. *Reporting of Injuries, Diseases and Dangerous Occurrences Regulations (RIDDOR) 1986.* London: HMSO, 1986.
45. Jenkins R. *Defining the problem: stress, depression and anxiety: causes, prevalence and consequences.* In: Jenkins R, Warman D, eds. *Promoting mental health policies in the workplace.* London: HMSO, 1993.
46. Macbride A, Lancee W, Freeman SJJ. The psychosocial impact of a labour dispute. *J Occup Psychol* 1981; **54:** 125-33.
47. Cox T. *Stress research and stress management: putting theory to work.* London: Health and Safety Executive, 1993 (HSE Contract Research Report 61/1993).
48. Department of Health. *A guide to mental health in the workplace.* London: Department of Health, 1993.
49. Department of Health. *ABC of mental health in the workplace.* London: Department of Health, 1994.
50. Health and Safety Executive. *Health aspects of job placement and rehabilitation: advice to employers.* London: HMSO, 1989 (HSE Guidance note; HS23).
51. Kettle M, Massie B. *Employer's guide to disabilities, 2nd edn.* Cambridge: Woodhead-Faulkener, 1986.
52. Faculty of Occupational Medicine, Royal College of Physicians of London. *Guidance on the ethics for occupational physicians, 4th edn.* London: Royal College of Physicians, 1993.
53. Stevens A, Raftery J, eds. *Health care needs assessment: the epidemiologically based needs assessment reviews (vols I and II).* Oxford: Radcliffe Press, 1994.
54. Department of Health. *On the State of the Public Health: the annual report of the Chief Medical Officer of the Department of Health for the year 1992.* London: HMSO, 1993; 109-10.
55. Department of Health. *On the State of the Public Health: the annual report of the Chief Medical Officer of the Department of Health for the year 1993.* London: HMSO, 1994; 115.
56. Department of Health, Welsh Office, Scottish Office Home and Health Department, Northern Ireland Department of Health and Social Security. *Report on Confidential Enquiries into Maternal Deaths in the United Kingdom 1988-90.* London: HMSO, 1994.
57. Department of Health. *Population health outcome indicators for the NHS: 1993: England: a consultation document.* London: Department of Health, 1993.
58. Audit Commission. *A prescription for improvement: towards more rational prescribing in general practice.* London: Audit Commission, 1994.
59. Clinical Standards Advisory Group. *Clinical Standards Advisory Group report on diabetes mellitus.* London: Department of Health, 1994.
60. *Chiropractors Act 1994.* London: HMSO, 1994.
61. Steering Committee of the Confidential Inquiry into Homicides and Suicides by Mentally Ill People. *A preliminary report on homicide.* London: Confidential Inquiry into Homicides and Suicides by Mentally Ill People, 1994.
62. Department of Health. *The Health of the Nation Key Area Handbook: mental illness, 2nd edn.* London: HMSO, 1994.
63. Department of Health. *Report of the Working Group on High Security and Related Psychiatric Provision.* London: Department of Health, 1994.
64. Department of Health, Home Office. *Report of the Department of Health and Home Office Working Group on Psychopathic Disorder.* London: Department of Health, 1994. Chair: Dr John Reed.
65. *Mental Health Act 1983.* London: HMSO, 1983.
66. Department of Health. *Changing Childbirth: part 1: report of the Expert Maternity Group.* London: HMSO, 1993. Chair: Baroness Cumberlege.
67. Human Fertilisation and Embryology Authority. *Third annual report.* London: Human Fertilisation and Embryology Authority, 1994.
68. Human Fertilisation and Embryology Authority. *Donated ovarian tissue in embryo research and assisted conception: public consultation document.* London: Human Fertilisation and Embryology Authority, 1994.
69. Department of Health. *Expert Group to investigate cot death theories.* London: Department of Health, 1994 (Press Release: H94/553).
70. Department of Health. *Paediatric intensive care.* Heywood (Lancashire): Department of Health, 1994 (Executive Letter: EL(94)10).
71. Department for Education, Welsh Office. *Code of practice on the identification and assessment of special educational needs.* London: Central Office of Information, 1994.
72. Department for Education, Department of Health. *The education of children with emotional and behavioural difficulties.* London: Department for Education, Department of Health, 1994 (DFE Circular: 9/94, DH Local Authority Circular: LAC(94)9).

73. Department for Education, Department of Health. *The education of sick children.* London: Department for Education, Department of Health, 1994 (DFE Circular: 12/94, DH Local Authority Circular: LAC(94)10, Health Service Guidelines: HSG(94)24).

74. Department for Education, Department of Health. *The education of children being looked after by Local Authorities.* London: Department for Education, Department of Health, 1994 (DFE Circular: 13/94, DH Local Authority Circular: LAC(94)11).

75. Department of Health. *Relieving the pressure: your guide to pressure sores.* Heywood (Lancashire): Department of Health, 1994.

76. Department of Health. *Report of the brain injury rehabilitation conference, Peterborough, March 1994.* Heywood (Lancashire): Department of Health, 1994.

77. UK Health Departments. *AIDS-HIV infected health care workers: guidance on the management of infected health care workers.* Heywood (Lancashire): Department of Health, 1994 (Health Service Guidelines: HSG (94)16).

78. Department of Health. *Offering voluntary named HIV antibody testing to women receiving antenatal care.* Heywood (Lancashire): Department of Health, 1994 (Professional Letter: PL/CO(94)3).

79. Hospital Infection Society, British Society for Antimicrobial Chemotherapy. Revised guidelines for the control of epidemic methicillin-resistant *Staphylococcus aureus.* *J Hosp Infect* 1990; **16:** 351-77.

80. NHS Executive. *Improving the effectiveness of NHS.* Heywood (Lancashire): Department of Health, 1994 (Executive Letter: EL(94)74).

81. Department of Health. *Clostridium difficile infection: prevention and management: a report by a Department of Health/Public Health Laboratory Service Joint Working Group.* Heywood (Lancashire): Department of Health, 1994.

82. Medical Research Council Institute for Environment and Health. *Air pollution and health: understanding the uncertainties.* Norwich: Institute for Environment and Health, 1994.

83. Medical Research Council Institute for Environment and Health. *Air pollution and respiratory disease: UK research priorities.* Norwich: Institute for Environment and Health, 1994.

84. House of Commons. Parliamentary Debate. Childhood Cancer, Dounreay. *Hansard* 19 July 1994; **247:** Col 120-1.

85. Department of Health. *Management of outbreaks of foodborne illness.* London: Department of Health, 1994.

86. Department of Health. Adverse reactions to alternative remedies. *CMO's Update* 1994; **4**: 2.

87. Ministry of Agriculture, Fisheries and Food Advisory Committee on Pesticides. *Advisory Committee on Pesticides Annual Report (1994).* London: HMSO, 1994.

88. *Pesticides (Maximum Residue Levels in Crops, Food and Feeding Stuffs) Regulations 1994.* London: HMSO, 1994 (Statutory Instrument: SI 1994 no. 1985).

89. Ministry of Agriculture, Fisheries and Food, Health and Safety Executive. *Annual Report of the Working Party on Pesticide Residues 1993.* London: HMSO, 1994.

90. Newton T, Grabham AH, Roberts G. *Hospital medical staffing: achieving a balance: plan for action: a report issued by the steering group for implementation on behalf of the Health Departments, the Joint Consultants Committee and the Chairmen of Regional Health Authorities.* London: Department of Health and Social Security, 1987.

91. Department of Health. *Hours of work of doctors in training: the new deal.* London: Department of Health, 1991 (Executive Letter: EL(91)82).

92. Department of Health. *Hospital doctors: training for the future: the report of the working group on specialist medical training.* London: Department of Health, 1993. Chair: Dr Kenneth Calman.

93. Department of Health. *Medical and dental staffing: centrally funded part-time consultants scheme.* Heywood (Lancashire): Department of Health, 1994 (Executive Letter: EL(94)42).

94. Department of Health. *Assimilation of Senior Clinical Medical Officers and Clinical Medical Officers into a combined child health service.* Heywood (Lancashire): Department of Health, 1994 (Health Service Guidelines: HSG(94)10).

95. House of Commons. Parliamentary Debate. Debate on the Address (Department of Health). *Hansard* 16 November 1994; **250**: Col 34.

96. *Medical Act 1983.* London: HMSO, 1983.

97. General Medical Council. *Proposed changes to the Medical Act 1983 to improve the working of the GMC's conduct and health procedures.* London: General Medical Council, 1992.

98. *The Medicines (Products Other Than Veterinary Drugs)(Prescription Only) Amendment (No. 2) Order 1994* London: HMSO, 1994 (Statutory Instrument: SI 1994 no. 3016).

99. Department of Health. *Standards for Local Research Ethics Committees: a framework for ethical review.* London: Department of Health, 1994.

100. House of Lords. Select Committee on Medical Ethics. *Report of the Select Committee on Medical Ethics: Volume 1: 1994.* London: HMSO, 1994. Chair: Baron Walton of Detchant.

101. Department of Health. *Government response to the report of the Select Committee on Medical Ethics.* London: HMSO, 1994 (Cm. 2553).

102. Office of Public Service and Science. *Realising Our Potential: a strategy for science, engineering and technology.* London: HMSO, 1993 (Cm. 2250).

103. Cabinet Office, Office of Public Service and Science, Office of Science and Technology. *Forward Look of Government funded science, engineering and technology.* London: HMSO, 1994.

104. NHS Management Executive. *Research and development in the new NHS: functions and responsibilities.* Leeds: Department of Health, 1994.

105. Research and Development Task Force. *Supporting research and development in the NHS.* London: HMSO, 1994. Chair: Professor Anthony Culyer.
106. Department of Health. *An oral health strategy for England.* London: Department of Health, 1994.
107. Department of Health. *Improving NHS dentistry.* London: HMSO, 1994 (Cm. 2625).
108. Todd J, Lader D, Dodd T. *Dental crowns: report of a follow-up to the 1988 adult health survey.* London: HMSO, 1994.
109. Todd J, Lader D. *Adult dental health: United Kingdom 1988.* London: HMSO, 1991.
110. *The Public Health (International Trains) Regulations 1994.* London: HMSO, 1994 (Statutory Instrument: SI 1994 no. 311).
111. *The Public Health (International Trains) Regulations 1994 (as amended by Statutory Instrument: SI 1994/1405).* London: HMSO, 1994 (Statutory Instrument: SI 1994 no. 1405).

Communications from the Chief Medical Officer to the medical profession and others during 1994

(Copies of Chief Medical Officer Letters and *CMO's Update* can be obtained from the Health Publications Unit, no. 2 site, Manchester Road, Heywood, Lancashire OL10 2PZ.)

CMO Letters

Report on the Confidential Enquiries into Maternal Deaths in the United Kingdom 1988-1990. (Professional Letter: PL/CMO(94)1) (16 January).
Meningococcal infection: meningitis and septicaemia. (Professional Letter: PL/CMO(94)2) (3 February).
Communications with the profession. (Professional Letter: PL/CMO(94)3) (22 February).
Treatment of depression in primary care: effective health care bulletin. (Professional Letter: PL/CMO(94)4) (1 March).
Hospital doctors: training for the future: implementation of the report. (Professional Letter: PL/CMO(94)5) (14 March).
Quality in the cervical cancer screening programme: professional guidance and training. (Professional Letter: PL/CMO(94)6) (30 March).
Quality assurance in radiotherapy. (Professional Letter: PL/CMO(94)7) (3 May).
Termination of pregnancy by medical methods: the role of the registered nurse or midwife and others who are not registered medical practitioners. (Professional Letter: PL/CMO(94)8) (24 June).
Standing Medical Advisory Committee: report on the management of lung cancer: current clinical practices. (Professional Letter: PL/CMO(94)9) (5 July).
National measles and rubella immunisation campaign (Professional Letter: PL/CMO(94)10) (28 July).
Influenza vaccine. (Professional Letter: PL/CMO(94)11) (20 September).
Measles and rubella immunisation campaign. (Professional Letter: PL/CMO(94)12) (27 September).
Update on national measles/rubella immunisation campaign. (Professional Letter: PL/CMO(94)13) (19 December).

CMO's Update

CMO's Update 1 (January). Includes: Effective Health Care bulletins; Health of the Nation; Asplenic patients and immunisation; Breast Implant Registry; CMO's Annual Report; Hepatitis B: protection of health care workers and patients; 1991 Health Survey for England; Notification of termination of pregnancy.

CMO's Update 2 (May). Includes: Immunisation update; Air pollution: oxides of nitrogen; Corticosteroids and varicella-zoster virus; Health effects of passive smoking; Screening policy in the NHS; Peanut anaphylaxis; HIV/AIDS: the issues; Breast implants and breast-feeding; Maternal deaths; sheep dips; Healthy holidays.

CMO's Update 3 (June). Includes: Influenza immunisation; Discharge guidance for people with mental illness; Antibiotic therapy in immunosuppressed people; Health on holiday.

CMO's Update 4 (November). Includes: New national thesaurus; Adverse reactions to alternative remedies; Hepatitis B: NHS Injury Benefits Scheme; TOXBASE for poisons; Supply of single-dose oral poliomyelitis vaccine; Management of lung cancer; Sickle cell, thalassaemia and other haemoglobinopathies; Safe use of diagnostic ultrasound; Obstetric cholestasis; HoNOS: a psychiatric thermometer; Public health LINK; On the State of the Public Health 1993; Health of adolescents.

Public health LINK

The urgent electronic and facsimile (fax) cascade messaging system was used for the first time during 1994 (see page 59) and copies of the following messages can be obtained from the Chief Medical Officer, Department of Health, Richmond House, 79 Whitehall, London, SW1A 2NS.

Public health LINK: test message (Cascade Electronic Message: CEM/CMO(94)1) (6 July).
Plague in India (Cascade Electronic Message: CEM/CMO(94) 2) (28 September).
Plague in India (Cascade Electronic Message: CEM/CMO(94)3) (5 October).
Warning on the use of face paints (Cascade Electronic Message: CEM/CMO(94)4) (31 October).

CHAPTER ONE

VITAL STATISTICS

(a)   Population size

The estimated resident population of England at 30 June 1994 was 48.7 million, an increase of 175,000 (0.4%) compared with 1993. There was natural increase (the excess of births over deaths) of approximately 100,000 and net inward migration of some 74,000 between mid-1993 and mid-1994.

(b)   Age and sex structure of the resident population

Appendix Table A.1 shows how the sizes of populations in various age-groups have changed in the period 1981-91 and in each of the three years 1991-92, 1992-93 and 1993-94. The number of children below school age (0-4 years) has remained fairly stable in recent years. The population of children of school age (5-15 years) is now increasing slowly, after falling during the 1980s. The relatively small late-1970s birth cohorts are now entering the youngest working age-group (16-29 years), the size of which is consequently declining. Larger cohorts born in the period after World War II, up to and including the 1960s, are now in the older working age-groups (30-64 years for men and 30-59 years for women), which are increasing in size. Numbers in the youngest pensioner age-group (65-74 years for men and 60-74 years for women) remain stable. Those aged 75-84 years have fallen slightly in number as survivors from the small cohorts born during World War I have reached this age-group. The most elderly group (aged 85 years and over) continues to increase rapidly and represents a growing proportion of all pensioners. About two-thirds of persons above pensionable age (65 years for men and 60 years for women), and three-quarters of those aged 85 years and over, are women.

Expectation of life at birth is estimated to be 74.2 years for males and 79.6 years for females born in 1994 in England and Wales, compared with 71.9 years and 77.8 years, respectively, in 1984, and 52.8 years and 56.1 years, respectively, in 1919, when the then Ministry of Health was established.

(c)   Fertility statistics - aspects of relevance for health care

Total conceptions

Data on conceptions relate to pregnancies which led to a maternity or to a legal termination under the Abortion Act 1967[1,2]; they exclude spontaneous and illegal abortions. The development of new computer systems has resulted in delays to some births and abortions data. The latest available conceptions data are for 1992, when 785,000 conceptions occurred to women resident in England, a fall of 3% from 1991 (see Table 1.1). The overall conception rate in 1992 was 76.4 per 1,000 women aged 15-44 years.

Table 1.1: *Conceptions by outcome, England, 1987, 1991 and 1992*

Age of woman	1987 †	1991	1992
*Under 16 **			
Number (000s)	8.95	7.4	6.8
Rate			
Total	9.3	9.3	8.4
Maternities	4.2	4.5	4.1
Abortions	5.1	4.8	4.3
*Under 20 ***			
Number (000s)	115.7	96.9	87.3
Rate			
Total	65.8	64.8	61.4
Maternities	42.7	42.2	40.0
Abortions	23.1	22.6	21.4
*All ages ****			
Number (000s)	804.8	809.1	784.9
Rate			
Total	77.5	77.8	76.4
Maternities	62.7	62.6	61.5
Abortions	14.8	15.2	14.9

*   Rates per 1,000 females aged 13-15 years.
**   Rates per 1,000 females aged 15-19 years.
***   Rates per 1,000 females aged 15-44 years.
†   Rates for 1987 are based on revised mid-year population estimates, derived to be consistent with both the 1981 and 1991 Censuses.

Source: OPCS

Table 1.2: *Live births and proportion of live births outside marriage, crude birth rate, general and total period fertility rates, and sex ratio, England, 1984, 1993 and 1994*

Year of birth	Live births	Crude birth rate*	General fertility rate†	Total period fertility rate (TPFR)	Percentage of live births outside marriage	Sex ratio
1984	600573	12.8	59.6	1.75	17.4	104.9
1993	636473	13.1	62.5	1.76	32.0	105.6
1994	628956	13.0‡	61.8‡	1.73‡	32.2	105.6

* Births per 1,000 population of all ages.
† Births per 1,000 females aged 15-44 years.
‡ Provisional.
Sex ratio represents number of male births per 100 female births.

Source: OPCS

Total births

Table 1.2 shows there were 628,956 live births in 1994 in England, 1% fewer than in 1993. This was the fourth successive year to show a decrease, and followed a fall of over 2% between 1992 and 1993.

The total period fertility rate (TPFR) measures the average number of children that would be born per woman if the current age-specific fertility rates continued throughout her childbearing years. It was 1.76 in 1993, compared with 1.79 in 1992. Since 1972, the TPFR for England has remained below 2.1, the level which would lead to the long-term 'natural' replacement of the population.

Whilst the overall number of live births decreased, the proportion which occurred outside marriage increased between 1992 and 1993 by 1% to 32% of all births. The proportion of births outside marriage remained at 32% in 1994 - the first year since the mid-1970s in which this proportion has not shown a rise on the previous year. In 1993, over half of all births outside marriage were jointly registered by parents who were living at the same address, and presumably cohabiting.

Table 1.3: *Numbers and rates of live births to women aged 40 years and over, England, 1988, 1992 and 1993*

Woman's age (years)	Numbers of births		
	1988	1992	1993
40	3476	3813	4005
41	2290	2452	2605
42	1253	1591	1579
43	715	884	882
44	367	484	457
40-44	*8101*	*9224*	*9528*
45	181	251	236
46	101	96	106
47	62	43	49
48	58	24	31
49	24	15	16
45-49	*426*	*429*	*438*
50 and over	66	50	70
40 and over	8593	9703	10036
Rates per 1,000			
40-44	4.8	5.6	5.9
45-49	0.4	0.3	0.3

Source: OPCS

Table 1.4: *Maternities with multiple births by age of mother, England and Wales, 1983 and 1993*

Age of mother (years)	1983			1993		
	Total	Twins only	Triplets and over	Total	Twins only	Triplets and over
Numbers						
All ages	6387	6293	94	8549	8302	247
Under 20	312	311	1	286	283	3
20-24	1616	1597	19	1407	1393	14
25-29	2243	2208	35	2800	2716	84
30-34	1559	1527	32	2794	2693	101
35-39	592	585	7	1096	1054	42
40 and over	65	65	-	166	163	3
Rates per 1,000 maternities						
All ages	10.2	10.0	0.2	12.8	12.4	0.4
Under 20	5.8	5.7	0.0	6.3	6.3	0.1
20-24	8.4	8.4	0.1	9.3	9.2	0.1
25-29	10.5	10.4	0.2	12.0	11.6	0.4
30-34	13.0	12.7	0.3	16.5	15.9	0.6
35-39	14.4	14.3	0.2	18.9	18.1	0.7
40 and over	9.4	9.4	0.0	15.9	15.6	0.3

Note: Rates for women aged under 20 years and 40 years and over are based upon the population of women aged 15-19 and 40-44 years, respectively: total rates may not match sum of twins/triplets and over due to rounding.

Source: OPCS

Fertility of women aged 40 years and over

The trend in recent years to delay childbearing has led to increases in the fertility of older women. As well as higher fertility among women aged 30-39 years, more births per woman have occurred in older women: between 1988 and 1993, there was a 23% rise in the fertility rate among women aged 40-44 years (see Table 1.3). In 1993, women aged 40-44 years showed the third highest rate of multiple maternities after women aged 35-39 and 30-34 years (see Table 1.4), and this rate had increased by nearly 70% between 1983 and 1993 - the greatest increase for any age-group.

Conceptions to girls aged under 16 years

In 1992, the conception rate in England for girls aged under 16 years was 8.4 conceptions per 1,000 girls aged 13-15 years. During the period 1989-91, the conception rate for girls aged under 16 years varied greatly in District Health Authorities (DHAs) across the country: the highest rate was seen in North Manchester (19.9) and the lowest in Tunbridge Wells (3.6) (see Table 1.5). The rates quoted here are based on data smoothed over the three years because of the small annual numbers of conceptions to girls in this age-group in individual

Table 1.5: *District Health Authorities with highest and lowest conception rates among girls aged under 16 years, England, 1989-91*

Area of usual residence	Rates per 1,000 girls aged 13-15 years		
	Total	Maternities	Abortions
Areas with high rates			
North Manchester	19.9	13.8	6.1
South Manchester	16.4	11.0	5.3
Doncaster	15.7	7.4	8.4
Central Manchester	15.4	11.3	4.2
Grimsby & Scunthorpe	14.7	6.7	8.0
Areas with low rates			
Preston	9.8	7.1	2.7
Basingstoke & North Hampshire	5.7	3.1	2.6
Barnet	4.9	1.3	3.5
South West Surrey	4.4	1.0	3.4
Tunbridge Wells	3.6	1.2	2.4

Note: Boundaries as on 1 April 1993; rates based on data smoothed over the three years 1989-91.

Source: OPCS

DHAs. The Manchester DHAs had the greatest maternity rates (conceptions leading to maternities) at 13.8, 11.3 and 11.0 for North, Central and South Manchester, respectively. The lowest maternity rate occurred in South West Surrey (1.0). Doncaster and Grimsby and Scunthorpe had the highest abortion rates (conceptions leading to abortion) at 8.4 and 8.0, respectively. The lowest rate leading to abortion was in Tunbridge Wells (2.4 per 1,000 girls).

Abortions

Based on provisional data, a total of 149,640 abortions were performed in 1994 under the Abortion Act 1967[1,2] on women who were resident in England. This represents a decrease of 1,279 (1%) compared with 1993, but an increase of 19,489 (15%) compared with 1984. Of the total, 89% were carried out at under 13 weeks gestation, and only 3% were performed beyond 16 weeks gestation.

In 1994, 29% of all abortions carried out on resident women were on those in their early 20s, whilst only 13% were on those aged 35 years and over. The abortion rate was highest among women aged 20-24 years (24.6 abortions per 1,000 women aged 20-24 years).

In 1994, 18% of legal abortions were on women aged under 20 years; of these, 11% were on girls aged under 16 years. Over the past decade abortions on women aged under 20 years have risen from 16.2 per 1,000 women aged 14-19 years in 1984 to 16.3 per 1,000 in 1994.

References

1. *Abortion Act 1967.* London: HMSO, 1967.
2. *Abortion Act 1967 (as amended by Statutory Instrument: SI 480c.10).* London: HMSO, 1991.

45

(d)   Mortality

The number of deaths registered in England increased from 522,656 in 1992 to 540,554 in 1993, a rise of 3.4%, and then decreased to 516,095 in 1994, a fall of 4.5%. The crude mortality rate rose from 10.8 per 1,000 population in 1992, to 11.1 per 1,000 in 1993, and fell to 10.6 per 1,000 in 1994. All figures for 1994 are provisional.

1993 mortality data

The Office of Population Censuses and Survey (OPCS) recently carried out an extensive redevelopment of its collection and processing systems for events data - in particular, for births and deaths. For deaths, this process has included progressive computerisation of registration in local offices; the setting up of a large deaths database to hold all deaths data from 1993; and the introduction of automated coding of cause of death. As a result of these changes to the way in which deaths are coded, and some other factors (such as an absence of medical inquiries during 1993), 1993 mortality data for some causes of death may not be directly comparable with those for 1992 and earlier years.

Mortality rates 1984-94

Mortality rates among males and females fell throughout the 1980s for most age-groups (see Figures 1.1 and 1.2). However, the mortality rate for men aged 15-44 years rose by 7% between 1985 and 1990; since 1990, this rate has fallen by 9% (see Figure 1.1). Although there was a slight rise in the mortality rates among those aged 75 years and over in 1993, the 1994 mortality rates for this age-group fell by a similar amount, bringing the rates back down to the 1992 level. Mortality rates among children aged 1-14 years have fallen dramatically since 1988 - by 32% and 29% among boys and girls, respectively.

Suicides and undetermined deaths

A recent study[1] of suicides and undetermined deaths in England and Wales over the period 1982-92 indicates that easy access to effective means of death is an important factor in suicide mortality. Suicides in people aged 16-74 years were analysed by occupation (ten highest-risk occupations for men and women, and all occupations combined) and method.

For men in all occupations combined, poisoning by motor vehicle exhaust gas is the most common method of suicide, accounting for one-quarter of deaths. However, poisoning by solid or liquid substances is the method of suicide favoured by men in health-related professions, including medical practitioners (half of deaths), pharmacists (two-thirds), dental practitioners (one-quarter), veterinary surgeons (two-thirds), and chemical scientists and engineers (one-third). All these occupations have easy access to drugs and other harmful substances. Poisoning accounts for one-fifth of male suicides in all occupations combined. Firearms are the favoured suicide method among farmers, accounting

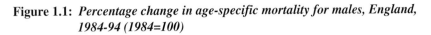

Figure 1.1: *Percentage change in age-specific mortality for males, England, 1984-94 (1984=100)*

Percentage

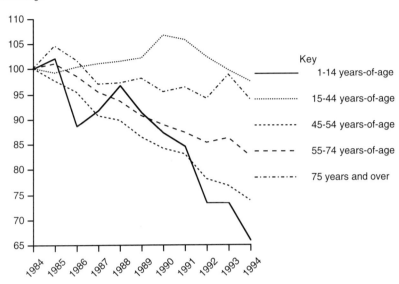

Source: OPCS

Figure 1.2: *Percentage change in age-specific mortality for females, England, 1984-94 (1984=100)*

Percentage

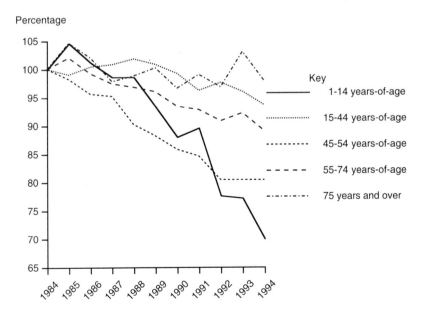

Source: OPCS

47

for 38% of deaths, compared with just 5% for all male suicides. Firearms are also used in 21% of suicides among veterinary surgeons and 15% of suicides in forestry workers - two other groups likely to have easy access to shotguns.

For women, poisoning by solid or liquid substances is the most common method, used in nearly half of all suicides. As for men, the use of poisoning is particularly high in health-related professions: pharmacists, nurses and medical practitioners use this method in 83%, 58% and 56% of suicides, respectively.

Reference

1.   Kelly S, Charlton J, Jenkins R. Suicide deaths in England and Wales, 1982-92: the contribution of occupation and geography. *Population Trends (in press).*

(e)   Prevalence of disease in the community

Morbidity statistics from general practice

Between 1 September 1991 and 31 August 1992, 60 general practices in England and Wales took part in the fourth of a series of studies of general practitioners (GPs) and their patients (MSGP-4)[1]. Nearly half a million patients were involved and socio-economic data were obtained for 83% of them. Details of each face-to-face contact with a patient were recorded, including the reasons for the consultation.

Practice morbidity surveys measure the illness recorded by the GP whom the patient consults; they do not measure total illness but do indicate the demands being made for health care. In the following analysis, the consulting rate is the rate per 10,000 population at which people consulted during the year with a specific diagnosis (or group of diagnoses). The first incidence is the rate of first-ever episodes of a disease, whereas incidence is the rate of first-ever plus subsequent new episodes during the year.

The overall consulting rate continued to increase, to a greater extent for women than for men, rising to 86% and 70%, respectively, by 1991-92 (see Figure 1.3).

Cancer

Consulting rates for all malignant disease increased from 68 per 10,000 in 1981-82 to 90 per 10,000 in 1991-92. The consulting rate for cancer of the larynx, trachea, bronchus or lung fell by 29% for males and rose by 25% for females (see Table 1.6). The consulting rate for cancer of the female breast increased by 30% during the same period. In men, the first incidence of lung cancer decreased by 33%, whereas in women the first incidence for both cancers increased above age 75 years and decreased below this age. The reduced prevalence and incidence of larynx, trachea, bronchus or lung cancer in males is likely to represent a true reduction in this condition, which is not shared by females. The unchanged overall first incidence but increased prevalence of breast cancer in females may represent increased survival following diagnosis.

Figure 1.3: *Consulting rates in general practice, England and Wales, 1955-56, 1970-71, 1981-82 and 1991-92*

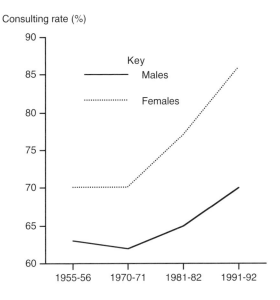

Source: OPCS, MSGP

Circulatory diseases

Consulting rates for circulatory diseases increased from 850 per 10,000 in 1981-82 to 931 in 1991-92. Table 1.7 shows small increases in consulting rates for uncomplicated hypertension (11% males, 7% females) and large increases for cerebrovascular disease (64% and 56%, respectively). Despite a large increase in consultations for angina pectoris (60% and 69%, respectively), there was a marked reduction in the prevalence of acute myocardial infarction of 31% among men and women alike.

First incidence of all these conditions was lower in 1991-92 than 1981-82. Overall incidence rates are falling, although more people are consulting doctors for treatment of angina and cerebrovascular disease. Acute myocardial infarction shows reduced prevalence and incidence. These results indicate that hypertension and angina may now be more effectively diagnosed and treated.

Mental disorders

Between 1981-82 and 1991-92, there was a reduction in consulting rates for mental disorders of 9% for males and 16% for females. The reductions were evident for anxiety states and depressive disorders, and seen across all age-groups. Serious disorders showed an increase in consulting rates from 72 to 113 per 10,000 without an associated increase in incidence.

Table 1.6: *Consulting rates per 10,000 person-years at risk for cancer of the larynx, trachea, bronchus or lung in males and females, and for female breast cancer, England and Wales, 1981-82 and 1991-92*

		Age (years)				
		All ages	25-44	45-64	65-74	75+
Cancer of larynx, trachea bronchus or lung						
Males	1981-82	14	2	24	66	66
	1991-92	10	1	16	51	67
Females	1981-82	4	0	10	18	7
	1991-92	5	0	10	17	17
Cancer of female breast						
	1981-82	23	8	44	72	69
	1991-92	30	10	61	81	88

Source: OPCS, MSGP

Table 1.7: *Consulting rates per 10,000 person-years at risk for selected circulatory disorders, England and Wales, 1981-82 and 1991-92*

		Age (years)				
		All ages	25-44	45-64	65-74	75+
Uncomplicated hypertension						
Males	1981-82	314	116	737	1149	754
	1991-92	347	100	757	1485	836
Females	1981-82	427	118	873	1477	968
	1991-92	459	96	867	1789	1127
Acute myocardial infarction						
Males	1981-82	55	16	117	199	224
	1991-92	38	6	73	158	186
Females	1981-82	29	3	38	111	128
	1991-92	20	1	20	71	118
Cerebrovascular disease						
Males	1981-82	39	2	42	153	396
	1991-92	64	3	72	272	579
Females	1981-82	43	1	26	125	332
	1991-92	67	4	46	177	496

Source: OPCS, MSGP

Chronic sickness

The General Household Survey (GHS)[2] is a continuous survey collecting information about 20,000 adults and 5,000 children in Great Britain each year. It provides two measures of chronic sickness. Firstly, people are asked whether they have any long-standing illness, disability or infirmity. Those who answer yes are then asked "What is the matter with you?", and then whether this limits their activities in any way. Acute sickness is measured by asking whether, in the two weeks before interview, people had to cut down on any of the things they usually do because of illness or injury. In 1993, 34% reported a long-standing illness, 20% a limiting long-standing illness and 14% restricted activity in the previous two weeks. Figure 1.4 shows trends from 1979 to 1994 for these three measures for males and females separately. The data are presented as three-year moving averages to smooth out year-on-year fluctuations. The prevalence of acute sickness has changed little. The prevalence of reported long-standing illness increased during the 1980s; towards the end of the decade the increase slowed, and then a slight fall occurred.

Figure 1.4: *Three-year moving averages of measures of morbidity from the General Household Survey, males and females, Great Britain, 1979-94*

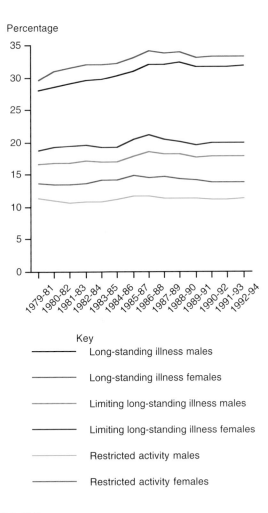

Source: OPCS, GHS

51

A question on long-term illness was also asked in the 1991 Census. The proportion of the population with a limiting long-term illness appears to vary among different ethnic groups, even when age-standardised to allow for different age structures[3]. Men and women of Bangladeshi and Pakistani origin reported particularly high age-standardised rates. Traditional industrial areas also tended to have high age-standardised rates of limiting long-term illness.

Health Survey data

The type of condition reported as the cause of long-standing illness was analysed by International Classification of Diseases (ICD) group in the 1989 GHS[2], and also in the 1991 and 1993 Health Surveys for England[4,5]. Illnesses associated with the musculo-skeletal system were most frequently mentioned as the cause of long-standing illness, followed by those affecting the heart and circulatory system and the respiratory system.

References

1. McCormick A, Fleming D, Charlton J. *Morbidity Statistics from General Practice: fourth national study: 1991-92.* London: HMSO (in press).
2. Office of Population Censuses and Surveys. *General Household Survey 1993.* London: HMSO (in press).
3. Charlton J, Wallace M, White I. Long-term illness: results from the 1991 Census. *Population Trends* 1994; **75**.
4. Office of Population Censuses and Surveys. *Health Survey for England 1991.* London: HMSO, 1993 (Series HS no.1)
5. Office of Population Censuses and Surveys. *Health Survey for England 1993.* London: HMSO (in press).

(f)   Infant and perinatal mortality

Provisional statistics for 1994 in England indicate that there were 3,842 infant deaths (babies who died under one year-of-age) compared with 3,995 in 1993. Of this total, 2,581 (67%) died in the neonatal period (under 28 days-of-age), and 1,261 (33%) in the post-neonatal period (between 28 days and 1 year-of-age). Thus the infant mortality rate fell by 3% between 1993 and 1994 to 6.1 per 1,000 live births, the lowest ever recorded (see Appendix Table A.5).

During 1994, there were 3,583 stillbirths in England, compared with 3,621 in 1993. The stillbirth rate remained steady at 5.7 per 1,000 total births (live births and stillbirths). One-quarter of these stillbirths were recorded as babies who died between 24 and 27 weeks gestation. (On 1 October 1992, the legal definition of a stillbirth was altered from a baby born dead after 28 complete weeks gestation or more to one born dead after 24 complete weeks gestation or more; comparisons with earlier years must take this change in legal definition into account.) The perinatal mortality rate (stillbirths and deaths of babies under 7 days-of-age per 1,000 total births) fell marginally from 8.9 in 1993 to 8.8 in 1994.

Appendix Table A.5 also shows that the post-neonatal mortality rate in England has fallen consistently every year since 1988; between 1988 and 1994, it fell by over 50% from 4.1 to 2.0 per 1,000 live births. Most of this fall can be accounted for by a 71% reduction in post-neonatal sudden infant death mortality rate (with a mention on the death certificate of 'cot death', sudden infant death syndrome [SIDS], or a similar term) over the same period. The highest annual fall in post-neonatal sudden infant deaths occurred between 1991 and 1992; between 1993 and 1994, the post-neonatal sudden infant death mortality rate in England remained unchanged at 0.6 per 1,000 live births.

Figure 1.5 shows infant mortality rates by the father's occupation (for births within marriage) for the period 1983-93. Babies of fathers in non-manual occupations had consistently lower mortality rates than babies of fathers in manual occupations.

Figure 1.5: *Infant mortality by father's occupational status, England, 1983-93*

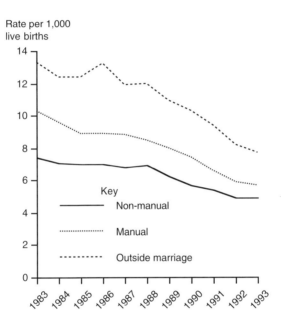

Source: OPCS

(g)   Trends in cancer* incidence and mortality

Data from the 1988 and 1989 GHS[1,2] show that 1% of adults reported cancer as a cause of long-standing illness. This estimate can be compared with that based on the OPCS Longitudinal Study, which is discussed in the report of the 1990 review of the cancer registration system[3]. The review brings together, for 1% of the population, information from the National Cancer Registration Scheme, successive Censuses and death registrations. It suggests that just over half a million people alive in 1981 would have had a cancer registered in the preceding ten years - again a prevalence of around 1%.

* cancer = malignant neoplasm

53

The latest national totals of cancer registrations relate to 1990. Appendix Tables A.7 and A.8 show the provisional numbers registered by age, sex and site; these are based on semi-aggregated data supplied by the regional cancer registries to OPCS. Although trends over the period 1979-90 must be interpreted with caution, for all malignant neoplasms (excluding non-melanoma skin cancer) there were increases of about 10% for males and over 15% for females. When specific sites of malignancy are examined there are some trends of note.

When adjusted for age, lung cancer registration decreased for males but increased for females between 1979 and 1990. For both sexes there were large increases in the number of registrations of malignant melanoma of the skin during the period 1979-90. During the same period the long-term decline in registrations of stomach cancer continued. There were marked downward trends for lymphosarcoma and reticulosarcoma and for Hodgkin's disease, but an upward trend for other malignant neoplasms of lymphoid and histiocytic tissue, to which less well-specified lymphomas would be coded.

There have been upward trends for cancers of the prostate, and kidney and other unspecified urinary organs between 1979 and 1990. As a result of a change in coding practice, the number of registrations of carcinoma-in-situ of the cervix uteri was very much higher in 1984 than in previous years. The numbers have continued to increase: in 1990, the total number of registrations was approximately double that in 1979. However, in respect of carcinoma-in-situ, possible improvements in the level of completeness of registration and in ascertainment need to be taken into account.

As with the incidence of all cancers, there has been no decline in all-cause mortality in recent years. Age-standardised death rates since the 1920s are shown in the 1992 Report[4]. For males, the post-war rise levelled off in the 1970s. For females, there was a declining trend until the early 1960s, followed by a rise. Within these totals, however, there was a rise and then a fall in the rate for cancer of the lung/bronchus in males, contrasting with a continuing rise in females. There was a steady fall in the rate for cancer of the stomach in both sexes. There has been a sharp decline in mortality from breast cancer since 1990.

References

1. Office of Population Censuses and Surveys. *General Household Survey 1988.* London: HMSO, 1990 (Series GHS no. 19).
2. Office of Population Censuses and Surveys. *General Household Survey 1989.* London: HMSO, 1991 (Series GHS no. 20).
3. Office of Population Censuses and Surveys. *Review of the national cancer registration system: report of the Working Group of the Registrar General's Medical Advisory Committee.* London: HMSO, 1990 (Series MB1 no. 17).
4. Department of Health. *On the State of the Public Health: the annual report of the Chief Medical Officer of the Department of Health for the year 1992.* London: HMSO, 1993; 44.

(h)   Trends in reporting congenital malformations

Appendix Table A.6 shows that, according to provisional data for 1994, the rate for malformed live births in England decreased to 69.2 per 10,000 live births,

17% lower than in 1993 and 39% lower than in 1990. The rate for malformed stillbirths increased to 2.4 per 10,000 total births, although this figure is 14% lower than in 1991 and 20% lower than in 1990.

An exclusion list was introduced in January 1990 to identify minor anomalies which should no longer be notified to OPCS. As a result, the total number of notifications received by OPCS fell by 4,058 (34%) between 1989 and 1990. This fall was accounted for entirely by a decrease in notifications of malformed live births. Three groups shown in the Table were affected by the exclusion list: ear and eye malformations, cardiovascular malformations and talipes. For these three groups the comments in the following paragraphs are restricted to the changes that took place between 1990 and 1994; for the remainder, the comments refer to changes between 1984 and 1994.

Since 1984, there has been a marked reduction in the rate of central nervous system anomalies for live births (from 9.9 to 2.5 per 10,000 live births) and stillbirths (from 2.7 to 0.7 per 10,000 total births). Conditions such as hydrocephalus and anencephaly, which are within the group most likely to be detected prenatally by diagnostic ultrasound or alphafetoprotein screening, have shown the largest fall. A similar decrease has been noted in other countries.

The rate of hypospadias/epispadias has approximately halved since 1980; in 1994, the rate was 7.2 per 10,000 live births. Since 1990, the rate of ear and eye malformations per 10,000 live births has fallen from 6.0 to 3.2 and that of talipes from 15.0 to 9.5. For cardiovascular malformations, the rate per 10,000 live births has decreased from 8.2 in 1990 to 5.5 in 1994, whilst the rate for stillbirths has remained at 0.3 per 10,000 total births.

(i)   **Appendix Tables and their content (pages 239-250)**

Appendix Table 1: *Population age and sex structure, England, mid-1994, and changes by age, 1981-91, 1991-92, 1992-93 and 1993-94.*

This Table is described on the first page of this chapter.

Appendix Table 2: *Five main causes of death for males and females at different ages, England, 1993.*

This Table contrasts the major causes of mortality in different age-groups. It should be noted that the rankings are dependent on the particular groupings of disease chosen. At the age of 35 years and over, the major burden of mortality derives from circulatory diseases and malignant neoplasms. At ages 15-34 years, road vehicle accidents, other causes of injury and poisoning, and suicide are major contributors to death, particularly among males. These causes of death - other than suicides - are also important in childhood, although congenital anomalies and diseases of the nervous system and sense organs also rank highly.

Appendix Table 3: *Relative mortality from various conditions when presented as numbers of deaths and future years of 'working life' lost, England and Wales, 1993.*

Data presented include the total number of deaths at all ages attributed to selected causes. The percentage distribution of the number of deaths demonstrates the major impact of circulatory disease and cancer in both sexes. In 1993, over 80% of deaths occurred at the age of 65 years and over.

Data are also presented for years of 'working life' lost between the ages of 15 and 64 years in order to indicate the impact of various causes of death occurring at younger ages. For this tabulation, a death occurring under the age of 15 years accounts for the loss of the full 50-year period between the ages of 15 and 64 years, whereas death at age 60 years contributes a loss of only 5 years of 'working life'. Thus weight is given to the age at death as well as the number of deaths, and emphasis is given to the burden of deaths occurring at younger ages.

For males, although circulatory disease and cancer still contribute substantially to loss of 'working life', other causes become more prominent. These include accidents (mainly motor vehicle) and suicide, and also those deaths occurring early in life - particularly infant deaths, which account for about 15% of years of 'working life' lost. Current registration procedures preclude presentation of infant deaths occurring under the age of 28 days in this table, although figures for sudden infant death syndrome (SIDS) - for which about 9% of cases occur under the age of 28 days - have been included.

For females, the total years of future 'working life' lost from all causes combined is much less than for males, relecting considerably lower death rates in females. Cancer - particularly of the breast, cervix, uterus and ovary - is a major contributor to loss of life in females aged under 65 years. In 1993, cancer accounted for 22% of all female deaths, but 45% of years of 'working life' lost. By contrast, although causing 45% of the total number of deaths, circulatory disease accounted for only 19% of the years of future 'working life' lost. In other respects, the pattern is broadly similar to that for males, although accidents account for a smaller proportion of deaths among females.

Appendix Table 4: *Trends in 'avoidable' deaths, England and Wales, 1979-93.*

The concept of 'avoidable' deaths was discussed in detail in the Report of 1987[1]. These indicators - developed in this country by Professor Walter Holland and his colleagues[2] - have been chosen to identify selected causes of mortality amenable to health service intervention, either preventive or curative. They might best be called 'potentially avoidable' deaths as, while it might not be possible to prevent every death deemed avoidable, it is expected that a substantial proportion could be prevented. The indicators are now published as part of the Public Health Common Data Set.

The Table presents recent secular trends of nine categories of 'avoidable' deaths. The data are presented as age-standardised mortality ratios, which adjust for differences in the age structure in the years compared. During the period 1979-93, substantial declines are evident in all of the categories presented. The age-standardised mortality ratio for all 'avoidable' deaths combined has fallen by more than 50% since 1979.

Appendix Table 5: *Live births, stillbirths, infant mortality and abortions, England, 1960, 1970, 1975-94.*

Trends are discussed in this chapter.

Appendix Table 6: *Congenital malformations, England, 1984, 1990, 1993 and 1994.*

Trends are discussed in this chapter.

Appendix Table 7: *Cancer registrations by age and site, males, England and Wales, 1990.*

The Table indicates the distribution of cancer registrations in men at different ages. At all ages combined, cancers of the lung, large intestine (including rectum) and prostate account for about half of the registrations. In childhood, a high proportion of cancers are attributable to leukaemias, lymphomas, tumours of the central nervous system, and embryonic tumours such as neuroblastomas and retinoblastomas. At older ages, cancer of the lung is the major cause registered. In the oldest age-group presented (85 years and over), prostate cancer accounts for slightly more registrations than lung cancer.

Appendix Table 8: *Cancer registrations by age and site, females, England and Wales, 1990.*

In childhood, the pattern of female cancers is broadly similar to that in males. However, in the 25-44 years age-group cancers of the breast (39%) and cervix (19%) predominate. At older ages, breast cancer continues to account for many registrations, although cancers of the lung and large intestine also occur in substantial numbers.

Appendix Table 9: *Immunisation uptake, England, 1980-93/94.*

The information presented in this Table is discussed in Chapter 6 (see page 171).

Appendix Table 10: *Cumulative total of AIDS cases by exposure category, England, to 31 December 1994.*

Recent trends in AIDS cases are discussed in Chapter 6 (see page 159).

Appendix Table 11: *Expectation of life at birth, all-cause death rates and infant mortality, England and European Community countries, circa 1992.*

This new Appendix Table includes two key overall measures of general health: expectation of life and infant mortality. Recent data are presented for each of the

European Community (EC) countries. Although problems often exist with regard to comparability of data, international comparisons provide an important perspective to the assessment of overall progress. In particular, such comparisons can highlight the scope for improvement and help to stimulate action to achieve progress.

In 1992, average life expectancy at birth in England and Wales was 73.9 years in males. Recent figures from our EC neighbours ranged from 70.6 years in Portugal to 74.7 years in Greece. The equivalent figure for females in England and Wales was 79.5 years, which compares with an EC range from 77.9 years in Ireland and Portugal to 82.0 years in France.

The infant mortality rate is also often used as a key descriptor of the overall health of a country. In 1992, the rate in England was 6.5 per 1,000 live births. This figure was one of the lowest in the EC at that time, contrasting with a rate in Greece in 1991 of 9.0. Nevertheless, there is no scope for complacency, with lower rates achieved in some other European countries (eg, 5.2 per 1,000 live births in Finland and Sweden and 4.8 in Iceland).

Additional information is presented on the age-standardised all-cause mortality rates for EC countries, with particular reference to deaths occurring under the age of 65 years. For males, the English death rate is well below the EC average and is only bettered by Greece and the Netherlands. However, for women the mortality rate is above average.

All international comparisons need to be made with some caution given possible differences in data collection and recording procedures. However, the indicators presented here are are among the most robust for the purpose of comparison.

Appendix Figure 1: *Weekly deaths, England and Wales, 1993 and 1994, and expected deaths, 1994.*

This Figure illustrates the week-by-week registrations of deaths from all causes at ages one year and over for 1993 and 1994. These can be compared with expected values for 1994 based on an average of deaths registered on the same week in the previous ten years, adjusted to allow for trends in death rates and in population.

References

1. Department of Health and Social Security. *On the State of the Public Health: the annual report of the Chief Medical Officer of the Department of Health and Social Security for the year 1987.* London: HMSO, 1988; 4, 72-82.
2. Charlton JR, Hartley RM, Silver R, Holland WW. Geographical variation in mortality from conditions amenable to medical intervention in England and Wales. *Lancet* 1983; **i:** 691-6.

CHAPTER 2

THE NATION'S HEALTH

(a)   Public health in England

In July, the Department of Health (DH) published *Public health in England: roles and responsibilities of the Department of Health and the NHS*[1]. This document set out a clear framework for the future in the light of changes in the Department's and the National Health Service's (NHS's) structure, and draws heavily upon the recommendations of the working party chaired by Dr Michael Abrams, formerly Deputy Chief Medical Officer[2]. This important report has been very well received and its significance widely recognised. The NHS Executive, for example, is using the implementation of its recommendations as one of the criteria by which the effectiveness of the new health authorities will be judged.

One of the main themes is to recognise the value of, and to support the contributions made by, people from a wide range of disciplines to improving the nation's health. The NHS Executive is committed to assisting the evolution of truly multidisciplinary public health departments in the NHS. As an example, publication of a report by the Standing Nursing and Midwifery Advisory Committee examines ways in which nursing, midwifery and health visiting practice in multidisciplinary public health work in the NHS might be developed[3].

The national Public Health Network continues to be the focus for the timely and accurate exchange of public health and medical intelligence among public health practitioners. Its function has been strengthened by the development of regional public health networks. Effective communications are essential to public health, and during the year two new ways of communicating information to doctors were introduced. In January, the inaugural issue of *CMO's Update* was published. This new publication supplements the long-standing system of Chief Medical Officer Letters (PL/CMO) and brings together several items which would otherwise have required individual Letters. Inevitably, the logistics of printing and distributing nearly 100,000 Letters takes several days, and there are occasions when a more timely messaging system is needed. It was for this reason that the urgent electronic and facsimile (fax) cascade system was introduced[4]. Over the last year it has been used to distribute urgent information about the plague in India (28 September and 5 October), and hazardous face paints (31 October) to general practitioners (GPs) and other doctors. It has also been used to provide timely information to directors of public health, for example about bovine spongiform encephalopathy; cot deaths; and the measles/rubella immunisation campaign. The urgent messaging system will continue to be developed in line with the NHS-wide networking strategy.

References

1. NHS Executive. *Public health in England: roles and responsibilities of the Department of Health and the NHS.* Leeds: NHS Executive, 1994.
2. Department of Health, Department of Environment. *Public health: roles and responsibilities of the NHS and roles of others.* Heywood (Lancashire): Department of Health, 1993 (Miscellaneous Circular: MISC(93)56).
3. Standing Nursing and Midwifery Advisory Committee. *Making it happen: public health: the contribution, role and development of nurses, midwives and health visitors.* London: Department of Health, 1994.
4. Department of Health. *Communications with the profession.* Heywood (Lancashire): Department of Health, 1994 (Professional Letter: PL/CMO(94)3).

(b)   Regional perspective

As a result of proposed legislation (subject to Parliamentary approval) from 1 April 1996, the configuration of health authorities as well as the central management of the NHS should be considerably streamlined. These changes will create new health authorities to replace the former District Health Authorities (DHAs) and Family Health Services Authorities (FHSAs). The legislation, if passed, will also abolish the eight remaining Regional Health Authorities (RHAs), with their strategic role being subsumed within Regional Offices of the NHS Executive (the body responsible for strategic management of the NHS in England).

The two years between Spring 1994, when these changes first began to take shape, and 1996, when they should be fully implemented, has been and will be hectic as NHS managers and health professionals discuss how change should be introduced. In times gone by, major NHS changes were perceived purely as reorganisations, with an emphasis on replacing one rigid structure with another. Typically, implementation was governed by detailed blueprints (for example, the 'Grey Book' of the 1974 reorganisation[1]). With the NHS reforms of 1990[2] and the proposed changes for 1996, a different approach has been taken. A strategic policy framework was created with considerable local flexibility as to the best ways in which services could be developed within it.

The role of public health medicine has been central to all these recent initiatives. First, the Health of the Nation strategy[3] has set goals and targets to improve the health of the whole population, which have become a focus for the strategic direction of the NHS as a whole. Second, a public health perspective will be at the heart of the work of the new local health authorities, with the proposal that directors of public health should be statutory members of the new authorities' boards. Third, public health is recognised as one of the key functions of DH and of the NHS Executive within it, with a proposal that a Regional Director of Public Health be appointed to each of the new Regional Offices of the NHS Executive.

The proposed public health component of the new Regional Offices will be a crucial element of the overall public health function within the NHS in England. Public health professionals, working locally in health authorities and NHS Trusts, will look to their Regional Office colleagues as the link with DH to brief them on important policy developments, for advice on implementation and to aggregate their local data on important issues and to feed this information back to the centre. Regional Directors of Public Health will continue to provide professional leadership and direction for the public health function as a whole, and co-ordination of effort on the many issues which overlap local population boundaries.

The eight new Regional Offices will be an important element in the revised management of the NHS, and an integral part of the NHS Executive; at the same time they should provide a close link with the people who actually see patients in geographical territories that cover very large areas.

Whilst detailed organisational structures will differ between Regional Offices, a number of general principles should apply. Most importantly, there should be a clear separation between staff who deal with functions related to the commissioning and purchasing of health care, and those whose functions relate to NHS Trusts. The first function will require the Regional Office to ensure the good performance of health authorities in areas of work such as meeting the needs of local populations, implementing national policy through contracting for health services, developing new ways of delivering primary care, and ensuring the development of the general practice fundholding programme. The second function will require monitoring the performance of NHS Trusts against their financial and non-financial duties and the review of proposals for capital investment.

The Regional Directors of Public Health and their teams of consultants in public health medicine and other public health professionals should all play a key role which does not place them on one or other side of the Regional Office structure described above. Rather, their public health expertise should have a wider influence to help to ensure the effective functioning of the new Regional Offices - partly through close working with management colleagues to enable public health measures to be fully integrated into the work of health authorities at local level. The public health role in Regional Offices should also ensure that public health expertise is appropriately brought to bear on the work of NHS Trusts. This is particularly important in the areas of clinical effectiveness, the use of information to assess outcomes of care and the development of critical appraisal skills among health care professionals. The public health team in the Regional Offices will also relate directly to counterparts in local health authorities and also (when asked to provide help and advice) to the medical directors of NHS Trusts. The proposals should ensure a clear link and effective co-ordination between the work of public health teams in DH and the NHS Executive, Regional Offices and local health authorities to ensure that important overall public goals to improve the health of the population and general medical care can be realised (see Figure 2.1).

Close working links will be maintained between Regional Office public health teams and academic departments and schools of epidemiology and public health. Through these links, the Regional Offices should help to shape postgraduate training in public health medicine, and to ensure that epidemiology and health services research appropriately address the needs of the service and that the

Figure 2.1: Organisation of the public health function in the NHS: impacts and interactions

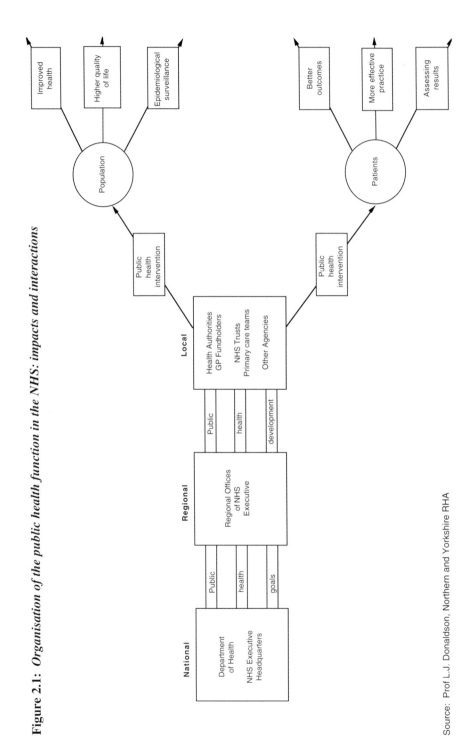

Source: Prof L.J. Donaldson, Northern and Yorkshire RHA

lessons from such research are acted on. In turn, the links (both formal and informal) with such academic institutions and their staff should bring additional expertise to the work of Regional Offices.

Over the past few years, the Chief Medical Officer has set up mechanisms to co-ordinate a network of public health expertise; this initiative has harnessed the many institutions and groups that ultimately contribute to the realisation of public health goals. The network enables information to be gathered, good practice to be shared, problems to be identified and solved, and new strategies to be devised.

The proposed changes are a logical consequence of the implementation of the *NHS and Community Care Act 1990*[4]. The underlying philosophy creates important opportunities for each part of the NHS to concentrate on a set of core responsibilities and emphasises the delegation of authority to take decisions as near as possible to where health care takes place. Regional Offices will be different to the old RHAs, in keeping with these principles. However, the scope and potential of the public health role within proposed new Regional Offices as part of a single focused central public health function will continue to be a major component of the NHS.

References

1. Department of Health and Social Security. *Management arrangements for the reorganised NHS*. London: HMSO, 1972.
2. Department of Health. *Working for patients*. London: HMSO, 1989 (Cm. 555).
3. Department of Health. *The Health of the Nation: a strategy for health in England*. London: HMSO, 1992 (Cm. 1986).
4. *NHS and Community Care Act 1990*. London: HMSO, 1990.

(c)   Inter-Departmental Group on Public Health

The Inter-Departmental Group on Public Health, chaired by the Chief Medical Officer in his role as Government Chief Medical Officer, facilitates inter-Departmental discussion and exchange of information on health issues. The Group usually meets three times a year to keep under review hazards to public health; to provide advice to Government on the assessment of such hazards; to provide an inter-Departmental forum for the discussion of scientific or technical issues that bear on public health; and to strengthen and to support existing links between other Government Departments and to identify and to correct any gaps in communications. The composition of the group reflects the public health interests of Government Departments[1].

Reference

1. Department of Health. *On the State of the Public Health: the annual report of the Chief Medical Officer of the Department of Health for the year 1993*. London: HMSO, 1994; 52.

(d)   Urban and rural differences in health

Concerns about the health of people who live in towns and cities is not a new phenomenon, but in recent times the possible consequences of a relative increase in urban populations in western and developing countries have been increasingly discussed. Urbanisation not only leads to an increased population density within a given geographical area, but influences means of governance and culture and alters the social and physical infrastructure[1]. International research into the health of people in cities, especially the urban poor, has identified a number of different factors which may contribute to poor health[2] - such as direct effects of low income or limited education; man-made conditions such as overcrowding and poor housing and sanitation; and the social and psychological consequences of urbanisation. The World Health Organization's (WHO's) 'Healthy Cities Project'[3] was launched in 1986 with collaboration between cities to develop local action plans for health promotion using community participation, together with a partnership between the public, private and voluntary sectors to focus on urban health.

Whilst up to now most attention has focused on the health problems of those living in urban areas, there may also be particular difficulties faced by those living in rural areas. Recent mortality data from the Office of Population Censuses and Surveys (OPCS) for 1990-92 indicate that mortality rates in rural areas are generally substantially lower than the national average, but exceptions include a slightly above-average mortality for deaths due to injury and poisoning (including accidents and suicides). Certain rural occupations are linked to specific types of mortality and morbidity: for example, the rate of suicide among farmers is nearly twice the average for all male occupational groups, which may reflect access to the means to commit suicide; attitude to death; and feelings of physical and social isolation. DH has taken a number of steps to tackle the high level of suicide among farmers, including support of the Samaritans' rural outreach initiative, and the production and distribution of a leaflet on the topic as part of the public information strategy on mental health.

The Fourth National Study of Morbidity Statistics from General Practice (MSGP-4)[4] also indicates that, except for older men, adults living in rural districts were about 10% less likely to consult for 'any reason' than those who lived in urban areas: in particular, fewer consultations related to preventive health measures were made by those aged 65 years and over in rural areas. A recent review by Watt and co-workers[5] has also highlighted the problem of service accessibility in rural areas.

References

1. Duhl L. *Healthy cities: myth or reality?* In: Ashton J, ed. *Healthy cities.* Milton Keynes: Open University Press, 1992; 15-21.
2. Harpham T, Lusty T, Vaughan P, eds. *In the shadow of the city: community health and the urban poor.* Oxford: Oxford University Press, 1988.
3. Davies JK, Kelly MP, eds. Healthy cities: research and practice. London: Routledge, 1993.
4. McCormick A, Fleming D, Charlton J. *Morbidity Statistics from General Practice: fourth national study 1991-92.* London: HMSO (in press).
5. Watt IS, Franks AJ, Sheldon TA. Health and health care of rural populations in the UK: is it better or worse? *J Epidemiol Commun Health* 1994; **48**: 16-21.

(e)   Variations in health

Significant variations in health may be observed in relation to geographical area, ethnicity, social class, occupation and gender. Such variations, which occur within England and internationally, present a challenge when their underlying causes can be identified and indicate potential for improvement. However, even when the reasons for such variations are known, it may be difficult to achieve improvement through health care interventions alone.

These problems can be illustrated if coronary heart disease (CHD) is used as an example. There are striking variations in CHD mortality within the population. Rates are higher in the north of England than in the south; higher among those born on the Indian sub-Continent but lower among those born in the Caribbean; higher among people in social class V than those in social class I; higher among those in manual than in non-manual occupations; and higher in men than in women[1].

Thus variations in health may be complex and inter-related, and causal factors may only be identified by careful assessment of all available evidence. Even when causes can be identified, the impact of interventions intended to reduce these variations may be unpredictable. The need for further scientifically based and well evaluated research has been recognised by the establishment of a sub-group of the Chief Medical Officer's Health of the Nation Working Group: this sub-group, which met for the first time in May and is due to submit a report during 1995, will focus on proposals for practical advice to the Department and the NHS to address health variations in the five Health of the Nation key areas[2].

During 1994, a new centre for Health and Society was launched at University College London Medical School. At the launch, Professor Michael Marmot and others presented data on health variations and their possible causes; the Chief Medical Officer also presented a paper on 'The potential of research on the socio-economic approach to prevention'. The British Medical Association (BMA) also held a conference on 'Social inequalities and health' and, at the European Health Policy Conference in Copenhagen in December, delegates agreed to pledge themselves to heighten people's awareness of the need for health policies and programmes that tackle inequities in health between different groups in the population.

References

1. Department of Health. *Coronary heart disease: an epidemiological overview*. London: HMSO, 1994.
2. Department of Health. *The Health of the Nation: a strategy for health in England*. London: HMSO, 1992 (Cm. 1986).

(f)   Substance misuse

Smoking

Trends in adult smoking prevalence by sex from 1974 to 1992 in England, and the projected reduction required to meet the year 2000 target, are shown in Figure 2.2. The figures show that adult smoking rates continue to fall: in 1992, some 29% of men smoked, compared with 31% in 1990; among women, 27%

smoked in 1992, compared with 28% in 1990. It cannot be assumed that current trends towards reduced smoking prevalence will necessarily continue, but so far encouraging progress has been made. Results from the 1990 Infant Feeding Survey[1] show that, in Great Britain, the number of mothers smoking cigarettes before pregnancy remained broadly static at 38%, while the proportion giving up smoking during pregnancy increased slightly from 24% in 1985 to 27% in 1990. Cigarette consumption in the United Kingdom (UK) dropped from 98,000 million cigarettes in the year to June 1990 to 84,000 million cigarettes in the year to June 1994.

The prevalence of regular cigarette smoking among 11-15-year-olds from 1982 to 1994 is set out in Figure 2.3 and Table 2.1. Statistics for 1994 indicate that regular smoking by all 11-15-year-olds has increased from 10% in 1993 to 12% in 1994, which is twice the Health of the Nation target. More girls than boys are regular smokers in this age-group, with rates of 13% and 10%, respectively. Some 28% of all 15-year-olds are regular smokers[2]. These results are disappointing, especially when set against progress towards the other smoking targets.

In February, the Government published *Smoke-free for health: an action plan to achieve the Health of the Nation targets on smoking*[3]. This document summarised the latest available evidence on the health impact of tobacco use, reported in detail on progress against targets and set out, for the first time, a comprehensive strategy to reduce smoking. March saw the first meeting of the Scientific Committee on Tobacco and Health. This Committee will report directly to the Chief Medical Officer on the health and behavioural aspects of tobacco use. On December 29, DH launched a three-year national smoking education campaign; this multi-media programme will cost £13.5 million and is aimed particularly at parents. Children whose parents smoke are twice as likely to smoke themselves than the children of non-smokers.

Alcohol

Patterns of alcohol consumption and drinking behaviour reported in the 1992 Health Survey for England[4] were broadly similar to those in the 1992 General Household Survey (GHS)[5]. About 30% of men and 13% of women drink more than the recommended sensible limits of 21 units per week for men and 14 for women. The survey also reports that among current drinkers, 9% of men and 5% of women said they had experienced at least two of a list of six physical or psychological problems associated with alcohol misuse and, as would be expected, the likelihood of problem drinking rose with the amount of alcohol consumed. Between 1991 and 1993, the Health Surveys for England show that overall alcohol consumption levels have not changed[4].

In recent years, a possible cardioprotective effect of alcohol consumption in relation to CHD has been suggested and has attracted considerable publicity. In August 1993, Mr John Bowis MP, Parliamentary Under Secretary of State for Health in the House of Commons announced the establishment of an Inter-

Figure 2.2: *Prevalence of cigarette smoking in adults (aged 16 years and over), England, 1974-92, with projection to health strategy target in 2000*

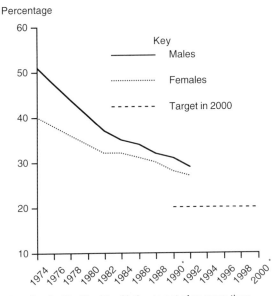

Percentage

Key
Males
Females
Target in 2000

Note: *Baseline for Health of the Nation target of no more than 20% of adults smoking cigarettes in year 2000.

Source: OPCS (GHS)

Figure 2.3: *Prevalence of regular cigarette smoking in children (aged 11-15 years), England, 1982-94*

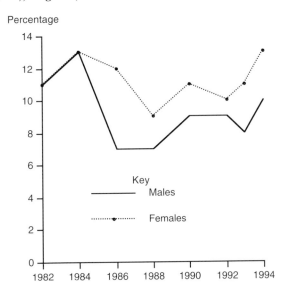

Percentage

Key
Males
Females

Source: OPCS

Table 2.1: *Prevalence of regular* cigarette smoking in children (aged 11-15 years), England, 1982-1994*

Year	Boys %	Girls %	Total %
1982	11	11	11
1984	13	13	13
1986	7	12	10
1988	7	9	8
1990	9	11	10
1992	9	10	10
1993	8	11	10
1994†	10	13	12

* Regular smoking defined as usually smoking at least one cigarette per week.
† Provisional data.

Source: OPCS

Departmental Group to review advice about sensible drinking levels in the light of current scientific evidence. The Group has received written evidence from a wide range of international experts and organisations and, following oral evidence, will report to Ministers in Summer 1995.

Drug misuse

The number of drug addicts notified to the Home Office in 1993 increased by 13% to 28,000, a slightly lower rate of increase compared with recent years. However, new addict notifications rose by 20% to 11,600, a similar increase to that in 1992[6]. In the six months to 30 September 1993, 16,810 individual drug misusers presented to services for treatment[7]: three-quarters were men, and 54% of all drug misusers were aged 20-29 years; heroin users accounted for 46%, methadone users 18% and amphetamine users 11% of the total.

In April, Dr Brian Mawhinney, then Minister for Health, announced the establishment of a Task Force to review services for drug misusers. The Task Force is conducting a comprehensive survey of clinical and operational aspects and the cost-effectiveness of existing services for drug misusers. It will report to Ministers in early 1996.

In October, the Government published its Green Paper, *Tackling Drugs Together*[8], to help to provide better co-ordination of policy and services at national and local levels. This important initiative has undergone widespread consultation and a White Paper is likely to be published in 1995.

References

1. White A, Freeth S, O'Brien M. *Infant feeding 1990: a survey carried out by the Social Survey Division of OPCS.* London: HMSO, 1992.
2. Office of Population Censuses and Surveys. *Smoking among secondary school children in England in 1994: an enquiry carried out by the Social Survey Division of OPCS on behalf of the Department of Health.* London: HMSO (in press).

3. Department of Health. *Smoke-free for health: an action plan to achieve the Health of the Nation targets on smoking.* Heywood (Lancashire): Department of Health, 1994.
4. Office of Population Censuses and Surveys. *Health Survey for England 1992.* London: HMSO, 1994.
5. Office of Population Censuses and Surveys. *General Household Survey 1992.* London: HMSO, 1994 (GHS no. 23).
6. Home Office. *Statistics of drug addicts notified to the Home Office, United Kingdom, 1993.* London: Home Office, 1994 (Statistical Bulletin 10/94).
7. Department of Health. *Drug misuse statistics.* Heywood (Lancashire): Department of Health (in press).
8. Lord President's Office. *Tackling Drugs Together: a consultation document on a strategy for England: 1995-1998.* London: HMSO, 1994 (Cm. 2678).

(g)   Nutrition

The Committee on Medical Aspects of Food Policy (COMA) published its report on *Weaning and the Weaning Diet* in October[1]. The report recommends that, for most infants, solid foods should not be introduced until 4 months-of-age and cow's milk as a main drink should be delayed until 12 months-of-age. Iron deficiency anaemia is considered in detail; particular issues which cause concern, such as vegetarian weaning and food allergies, are discussed; and the relation between nutrition in early life and adult health is explored.

COMA published its report *Nutritional aspects of cardiovascular disease*[2] in November. The Committee reviewed the latest scientific evidence that related diet to cardiovascular disease and made recommendations to reduce the population's risk of heart disease and stroke - which included a reduction in saturated fatty acid and total fat intakes, the eating of more starchy foods and fruit and vegetables, a reduction in average daily sodium intake, and the eating of oily fish at least every week.

In March, the Nutrition Task Force (NTF) published its action programme *Eat Well!*[3] to help to achieve the Health of the Nation nutrition targets, and set up project teams to implement its proposals. The NTF's leaflet *Healthy catering practice*[4], published in 1993 in collaboration with the Hotel Catering and Industrial Management Association, was disseminated. In June, a management handbook for the NHS[5] was produced to help purchasers and providers to identify actions to help to meet nutrition targets. The handbook was complemented by information produced in collaboration with the British Dietetic Association[6] to give examples of how dietitians can contribute in Health of the Nation key areas. In July, following wide consultation, a national food guide[7] was launched as a common basis for health professionals to educate people about a healthy, balanced diet. In November, a core nutrition curriculum document[8] designed to help those involved in health professionals' education to include nutrition in their courses was launched at a conference attended by 50 senior representatives of medical and nursing Royal Colleges and other health professional bodies.

Publicity material was produced for National Breastfeeding Awareness Week and the Department continued to support breastfeeding voluntary groups.

After a successful feasibility study, fieldwork began in October for a dietary survey of people aged 65 years or over, part of the National Diet and Nutrition Survey (NDNS) programme, sponsored by the Ministry of Agriculture, Fisheries and Food (MAFF) and DH. Fieldwork for the NDNS Survey of Children aged 1 to 4 years was completed and the report will be published in Spring 1995. A survey of infant feeding among Asian communities started in September.

Following the commissioning in 1993 of the first eight research projects under the auspices of the DH/Medical Research Council Nutrition Programme Committee[9], a meeting was held in June to identify and to develop future priorities for the programme; a report is expected in 1995.

References

1. Department of Health. *Weaning and the weaning diet: report of the Working Group on the Weaning Diet of the Committee on Medical Aspects of Food Policy.* London: HMSO, 1994 (Report on Health and Social Subjects; no. 45).
2. Department of Health. *Nutritional aspects of cardiovascular disease: report of the Cardiovascular Review Group.* London: HMSO, 1994 (Report on Health and Social Subjects; no. 46).
3. Department of Health. *Eat Well! An action plan from the Nutrition Task Force to achieve the Health of the Nation targets on diet and nutrition.* Heywood (Lancashire): Department of Health, 1994. Chair: Professor Dame Barbara Clayton.
4. Department of Health. *Healthy catering practice.* London: Department of Health, 1993.
5. Department of Health. *Nutrition and health: a management handbook for the NHS.* London: Department of Health, 1994.
6. Department of Health. *Targeting practice: the role of State Registered Dietitians.* London: Department of Health, 1994.
7. Health Education Authority. *The National Food Guide: the balance of good health.* London: Health Education Authority, 1994.
8. Department of Health. *Nutrition: core curriculum for nutrition in the education of health professionals.* London: Department of Health, 1994.
9. Department of Health. *On the State of the Public Health: the annual report of the Chief Medical Officer of the Department of Health for the year 1993.* London: HMSO, 1994; 69.

(h)   Health of people in later life

DH has continued to promote work on sickness and disability prevention among older people in line with the national strategy for health[1] with extensive revision of *Health and well-being: a guide for older people*[2]. Research on healthy active life expectancy will be reviewed at a meeting in April 1995 to discuss implications of the findings of two pilot studies on the use of healthy active life expectancy measures.

During 1994, there was considerable public debate about equity of access to acute hospital services for older people and the provision of long-term care by the NHS. Ministers emphasised that every citizen, regardless of age, has the right to receive health care on the basis of clinical need. A report by the Royal College of Physicians of London, *Ensuring equity and quality of care for elderly people*[3] was published.

In response to concerns about responsibilities for and funding of the care of elderly people, draft guidance on NHS responsibilities for meeting continuing health care needs was issued for consultation in August. Responses from a wide range of health and local authorities, voluntary organisations and individuals were received. These comments were considered carefully and final guidance will be issued early in 1995. This guidance will make clear that the NHS has important responsibilities to arrange and to fund a full range of services to meet needs for continuing health care.

DH supported the development of the Royal College of Physicians' Research Unit and British Geriatrics Society's good practice guidelines for geriatric day hospitals[4], and plans to distribute a copy of these guidelines to all DHAs and Family Health Services Authorities (FHSAs).

References

1. Department of Health. *The Health of the Nation: a strategy for health in England.* London: HMSO, 1992. (Cm. 1986).
2. Department of Health. *Health and well-being: a guide for older people.* Heywood (Lancashire): Department of Health (in press)
3. Royal College of Physicians of London. *Ensuring equity and quality of care for elderly people: the interface between geriatric medicine and general (internal) medicine.* London: Royal College of Physicians of London, 1994.
4. Royal College of Physicians Research Unit. *Geriatric day hospitals: their role and guidelines for good practice.* London: Royal College of Physicians of London, 1994.

(i)   Health of black and ethnic minorities

The Report for 1991[1] drew attention to some of the differences in health and disease patterns seen among people from black and ethnic minority communities, and highlighted the difficulties in access to health services experienced by some ethnic groups.

The NHS Ethnic Health Unit

The NHS Ethnic Health Unit made £1 million available to fund innovative projects during 1994 and this opportunity will be repeated in 1995. The Unit's work is focused upon improving communication between local minority ethnic groups and health authorities, so that clearer input by ethnic groups will improve local services in secondary, primary and community care. The Unit is also working on ways to improve the use of information on ethnic health by the NHS, and on the implementation of ethnic monitoring (see below).

Surveys and research

The Fourth National Survey of Ethnic Minorities is a survey of economic and social conditions of Britain's largest ethnic groups, conducted by the Policy Studies Institute, which for the first time contains sections on physical and mental health. The Health Education Authority's (HEA's) Health and Lifestyles Survey on Black and Ethnic Minorities will be published in 1995. DH has funded a number of projects related to the health of black and ethnic minorities in the five Health of the Nation key areas[2]. These include a study of severe mental illness amongst black subjects by the Royal Free Hospital[3].

71

Policy development

The Standing Medical Advisory Committee working party report on sickle cell, thalassaemia and other haemoglobinopathies was published early in 1994[4] and was widely distributed.

Ethnic monitoring

DH published national implementation guidance and training material entitled *Collecting ethnic group data for admitted patient care*[5]. This guidance was based on findings from national pilot sites and local initiatives together with consultative exercises with national, professional and public organisations including the medical and other professional Royal Colleges. The Department has funded the Office for Public Management to produce advice on developing a responsive health service and achieving equality in purchasing and provision, which will be published early in 1995. DH has also funded the Royal College of General Practitioners to undertake a study to improve the quality of general practitioner (GP) consultations for patients from ethnic minority communities.

Equal opportunities for NHS staff

The NHS Executive has continued to monitor and to support implementation of the programme of action for ethnic minority NHS staff, launched by Secretary of State for Health in December 1993. Ethnic monitoring data on the entire NHS workforce was collected for the first time in September 1994, and will be available in Autumn 1995. Progress towards implementation of the programme's goals will be monitored through reviews of performance management and business planning. £250,000 were made available to support implementation of the programme in NHS Trusts and health authorities in 1994/95, with a similar amount set aside for 1995/96.

References

1. Department of Health. *On the State of the Public Health: the annual report of the Chief Medical Officer of the Department of Health for the year 1991.* London: HMSO, 1992; 8-9, 54-77.
2. Department of Health. *The Health of the Nation: a strategy for health in England.* London: HMSO, 1992 (Cm. 1986).
3. King M, Coker E, Leavey G, Hoare A, Johnson-Sabine E. Incidence of psychotic illness in London: comparison of ethnic groups. *BMJ* 1994; **309**: 1115-9.
4. Department of Health. *Report of a Working Party of the Standing Medical Advisory Committee on sickle cell, thalassaemia and other haemoglobinopathies.* London: HMSO, 1994.
5. Department of Health, NHS Executive. *Collecting ethnic group data for admitted patient care: implementation, guidance and training material.* Leeds: NHS Information Management Group, 1994 (IMG C3025).

(j)   Health of men

The special chapter in the Report for 1992[1] examined the state of men's health and a brief update of progress was given in last year's Report[2]. Data now available show that while men's health continues to improve, it still lags behind that of women in many respects. Expectation of life at birth based on 1992 data is 74 years for men and 79 for women, compared with 71 years and 77 years, respectively, in 1982. Mortality from diseases such as CHD and stroke continue to fall, but much can still be done (see page 77).

Registration rates for cancer of the prostate were almost 30% higher in 1989 (the most recent year for which statistics are available) than in 1979. There was a substantial rise of 10% in registration rates between 1987 and 1988, but little change between 1988 and 1989. DH's Central Research and Development Committee Health Technology Panel has identified research into prostatic cancer as a high priority. Preliminary work has now started to assess cost-effectiveness and clinical benefit of different methods of screening for and management of prostate cancer.

Health and work

The importance of targeting men's health through their workplace was acknowledged in earlier Reports[1,2]. The results from three pilot projects referred to in last year's Report[2] have helped the Workplace Steering Group in its analysis of the best ways to develop health promotion in the workplace; a report is expected in 1995 and this topic is also discussed in Chapter 4.

Activities during the year

Increasing interest in the topic of men's health was seen during the year, including a major conference organised by the East Midlands Men's Health Network, which attracted considerable national media coverage. A health clinic specifically for men was established in Lewisham, South London, which is open in the evening and provides an opportunity for men to speak to male staff about all health matters.

In the report of Professor Roderic Griffiths, Regional Director for Public Health in West Midlands[3], the differences in health of men and women in the Region were examined. This highlighted, at a local level, much of what had been described earlier in the Chief Medical Officer's Report[1] and attracted considerable local interest.

A sub-group of the Chief Medical Officer's Health of the Nation Working Group was established to look at variations in health in the five key areas addressed in the health strategy[4], including socioeconomic, ethnic, geographical and gender variations. It will provide advice as to how DH and the NHS might make best use of existing information to tackle such variations and will also report on areas where further research is needed. The sub-group is expected to report to the Chief Medical Officer in 1995.

The way forward

Further work to promote men's health is planned for 1995, including a major two-day conference 'Men's Health Matters' in the Summer. New media interest in the topic following its identification in the 1992 Report will also help to build on current progress.

References

1. Department of Health. *On the State of the Public Health: the annual report of the Chief Medical Officer of the Department of Health for the year 1992.* London: HMSO, 1993; 79-106.
2. Department of Health. *On the State of the Public Health: the annual report of the Chief Medical Officer of the Department of Health for the year 1993.* London: HMSO, 1994; 57-58.
3. West Midlands Regional Health Authority. *Agenda for health: report of the Regional Director of Public Health.* Birmingham: West Midlands Health Authority, 1994.
4. Department of Health. *The Health of the Nation: a strategy for health in England.* London: HMSO, 1992 (Cm. 1986).

(k)   Health of adolescents

Last year's Report highlighted the health of adolescents[1], and its launch in September 1994 focused professional interest on health promotion among this age-group. Two one-day conferences to explore ways to use the skills of nurses, midwives and health visitors in adolescent health were planned for early 1995, and preparations started for various health promotion activities to target adolescents in 1995 and beyond. These include plans for a conference on the 'Health of the Young Nation' to mark the third anniversary of the Government's strategy for health[2].

In January, DH's Central Research and Development Committee established a multidisciplinary advisory group to advise on priorities for NHS research in mother and child (including adolescent) health; a consensus was reached in November and a report will be published in 1995. The advisory group gave top priority to several recommendations relevant to the health of adolescents - which included identification of the needs and views of young people on the appropriate delivery of services, especially primary health care. DH's central research programme has made research into adolescent risk behaviour a priority for 1995/96.

Various specific medical conditions and lifestyle factors relevant to the Health of the Nation[2] key areas highlighted in last year's special chapter are discussed in the chapters on the strategy for health (see pages 76-87) and health care (see pages 128-158),but certain issues merit additional emphasis. Inter-agency working is essential to ensure maximum access to young people - particularly when dealing with substance misuse and for the promotion of mental health, because young people with behavioural and emotional problems provide challenges for educational as well as health and social services. In 1994, DH and the Department for Education (DFE) published documents relevant to adolescent mental health (see page 9)[3,4]. Drug misuse (see pages 9 and 68) was the subject of a Government Green paper[5], published in October, and a draft circular published for consultation by DFE in November[6]. Smoking prevalence among young people is discussed on page 65. The Department of Employment is also collaborating with DH and DFE to improve advice on how young people's health might affect their career options. Pilot studies have been set up into voluntary schemes whereby 13-year-old children are invited to report persisting health problems so that health and careers staff may advise them on any implications for their choice of career.

References

1. Department of Health. *On the State of the Public Health: the report of the Chief Medical Officer of the Department of Health for the year 1993.* London: HMSO, 1994; 5, 74-112.
2. Department of Health. *The Health of the Nation: a strategy for health in England.* London: HMSO, 1992 (Cm. 1986).
3. Department for Education, Department of Health. *The education of children with emotional and behavioural difficulties.* London: Department for Education, Department of Health, 1994 (DFE Circular: 9/94; Local Authority Circular: LAC (94)9).
4. Department for Education, Welsh Office. *Code of Practice on the identification and assessment of special educational needs.* London: Central Office of Information, 1994.
5. Lord President's Office. *Tackling drugs together: a consultation document on a strategy for England 1995-98.* London: HMSO, 1994 (Cm. 2678).
6. Department for Education. *Drug prevention and schools.* London: Department for Education, 1995 (DFE Circular: 4/95).

CHAPTER 3

THE STRATEGY FOR HEALTH

(a)   Introduction

The Government's strategy for health in England, set out in the 1992 White Paper *The Health of the Nation*[1], is now well under way. The strategy emphasises the benefits and the importance of preventing ill health, as well as treating it. For this approach to be effective, all people must be encouraged, as far as possible, to take responsibility for their own health; in many areas, ultimate responsibility and ultimate benefit lie with the individual. But people cannot be coerced into living more healthily: education, information and empowerment are the tools at hand.

To focus attention most effectively it is necessary to have a small number of well-defined priorities. The strategy for health is therefore based on five key areas which account for large numbers of premature deaths; in which effective preventive intervention is possible; and where outcome can be measured. The targets set in these five key areas - coronary heart disease (CHD) and stroke; cancers; mental illness; HIV/AIDS and sexual health; and accidents - were intended to be challenging but achievable. Steady progress to date in most areas indicates that the targets were well designed, but a few areas stand out where movement is out of step with the timetable. For example, the 1995 target for gonorrhoea was achieved well ahead of time, whereas progress on targets for teenage smoking and obesity has been less encouraging and these areas are receiving special attention. Suicide rates fell by approximately 6% between 1993 and 1994.

Work continues to be taken forward across Government as a whole, with a special Cabinet sub-Committee, chaired by the Lord President of the Council, that continues to oversee implementation, monitoring and development of the strategy. There are also key committees based in the Department of Health (DH). Baroness Cumberlege, Parliamentary Under Secretary of State for Health in the House of Lords, chairs the Wider Health Working Group and oversees its sub-groups. The Chief Medical Officer's Working Group continues to oversee the monitoring of the health strategy and to review the more general public health and epidemiological issues concerned with its development; a sub-group is examining variations in health in the five key areas, with a specific remit to study evidence about the effectiveness of interventions and to make recommendations for future research. The membership and terms of reference of the Chief Executive's Working Group have been reviewed to reflect the structural changes in the NHS after its Functions and Manpower Review. The Group now advises the NHS Executive on implementation of the Health of the Nation strategy in and through the NHS.

Reference

1.   Department of Health. *The Health of the Nation: a strategy for health in England.* London: HMSO, 1992 (Cm. 1986).

(b)   Key areas and targets

(i)   *Coronary heart disease and stroke*

Action to achieve the CHD/stroke targets continued with specific initiatives to address the risk factors of raised blood pressure (and the associated risk of alcohol misuse), lack of physical activity, raised serum cholesterol and obesity (see page 69), and smoking (see page 65). CHD in women also received attention in 1994[1]: women appear to be less likely than men to receive coronary artery surgery[2] or thrombolytic therapy[3]. However, recent figures indicate that this difference may be reducing (UK Heart Attack Study, unpublished data). CHD among men is well recognised by public and clinicians alike; it is essential to ensure that stereotypes do not influence medical judgments or patients' attitudes[4], so that women can make equal use of available services.

The *Health Survey for England 1992*[5] again focused on cardiovascular disease and associated risk factors. However, the 1992 Survey also included measurements of plasma fibrinogen (a factor in blood clotting which is associated with CHD and stroke), and information about prescribed cardiovascular medicines, psychosocial factors and parental death from cardiovascular disease. The results showed that, among women, raised plasma fibrinogen concentration was associated with greater body-mass index, taking the contraceptive pill beyond the menopause and physical inactivity. A high proportion of people reported that a parent had died from a cardiovascular disease: for example, 20% of women reported this as the cause of death of their father, and 16% as the cause of death of their mother. The strongest psychosocial relation for cardiovascular risk factors was seen among inactive men, who were about twice as likely as those who were active to have a high General Health Questionnaire (GHQ) score (a measure of psychiatric disorders) and to perceive a severe lack of social support.

Two epidemiological overviews, on CHD[6] and on stroke[7], were published by DH's Central Health Monitoring Unit. These overviews bring together a broad range of up-to-date statistics on these diseases and their main risk factors for clinicians and other interested groups within and outside the Department.

The Health of the Nation Physical Activity Task Force, set up in 1993 to develop strategies for physical activity, continued to meet throughout 1994. It reviewed a number of areas including the scientific evidence for the health benefits of physical activity, particularly moderate activity; population groups with special needs; research issues; monitoring; and target setting. The Task Force considered national targets, but accepted that they might be counter-productive. A consultation document should be published in mid-1995. During 1994, the Physical Activity and the Nutrition Task Forces worked together to consider action aimed to prevent further increases in the prevalence of obesity.

CHD and stroke continue to be a focus of health promotion arrangements within the general practitioner (GP) contract. Almost 90% of GPs are running health promotion programmes which offer a full range of primary prevention related to CHD and stroke. In December, DH funded a conference at the King's Fund Centre to discuss the effectiveness of CHD prevention in primary care.

(ii)   Cancers

The Health of the Nation White Paper[8] focused on breast cancer, cervical cancer, skin cancer and lung cancer - four major cancers which accounted for about 35% of all cancer deaths in 1992.

Breast cancer

The National Health Service (NHS) breast screening programme is the linchpin of the strategy to achieve the target of a 25% reduction in breast cancer mortality in the population invited for screening by the year 2000 (from a 1990 baseline). All screening centres have completed their first round of screening and are now inviting women for their second screen after an interval of three years. Nearly a million women attend the NHS breast screening programme annually, which represents an uptake of 72% - slightly higher than the compliance target of at least 70%. In the first full round of screening, almost 15,000 cancers were detected by the programme in England, which is about 10% higher than the estimated target. The results of the screening programme continue to be closely monitored.

Cervical cancer

In 1993/94[9], 84% of women subject to call or recall within the national cervical cancer screening programme had been screened during the previous five and a half years. This coverage must be maintained, and the quality of the screening programmme must also be high: guidelines to assure the quality of the screening programme and to measure its effectiveness[10] were published by the National Co-ordinating Network. This Network, set up in 1988, also reported on the first five years of the full programme[11].

During the review of the management of the national programme, mentioned in last year's Report[12], DH recognised the need for a more formal mechanism of quality assurance. A full-time national co-ordinator was appointed in April to establish arrangements similar to those already in place for breast cancer screening.

Skin cancer

Achievement of the skin cancer target (to halt the year-on-year increase of skin cancer by 2005) will require individuals to be aware of the risks of ultraviolet (UV) exposure and thereby wish to change their behaviour, and for them to be able to do so within our social and economic environment. The Office of Population Censuses and Surveys (OPCS) established baseline measures of the public's knowledge, attitudes and behaviour regarding excessive sun exposure[13]. The Health Education Authority's (HEA's) 1994 'Sun Know How' campaign promoted the following main messages: avoid the mid-day sun; take care not to burn; and cover up and wear a hat. This campaign achieved wide media coverage and was awarded the Fleishman-Hillard award for writing excellence.

Information on ground-level UV radiation intensity and the risk of sunburn was made available for use by weather forecasters. Free advice on the risks of excessive sun exposure was provided both through the Health Information Service and through a 24-hour recorded message. Evaluation confirmed that, during 1994, 87% of adults were aware of some publicity about skin cancer and 51% saw the UV forecasts.

Lung cancer

Smoking remains by far the major risk factor for lung cancer, and five Health of the Nation targets relate to lung cancer and smoking issues (see page 65). OPCS figures for England and Wales in 1989 show that lung cancer was the most common cancer among males, accounting for one-quarter of all registrations of malignant neoplasms (excluding non-melanoma skin cancers), and the third most common in females, accounting for 11%[14]; the corresponding figures for cancer deaths in 1994 were 29% and 16%, respectively, and caused 6% of all deaths.

The incidence of lung cancer in males rises steeply with age from the mid-30s and exceeds 500 per 100,000 population in men aged 70-74 years, and exceeds 750 per 100,000 population in those aged 80-84 years; overall, the current incidence among women is about 45% of that in men[14].

Over the past decade there has been a fall in standardised registration ratios (SRRs) for lung cancer among men in England and Wales, which in 1989 were 15% below the level in 1979. By contrast, there has been a large increase in SRRs among women, although in 1989 there was an indication that this rate of increase may be slowing[14].

In August, the Standing Medical Advisory Committee produced a report on the management of lung cancer[15], which was sent to all general practices and to hospital practitioners with a major interest in the management of lung cancer[16].

(iii)   Mental illness

Considerable progress has been made during 1994 in developing strategies to achieve the targets set under the mental illness key area of the strategy for health[8].

The National Psychiatric Morbidity Survey[17], commissioned by DH and conducted by OPCS, produced the first definitive results to replace previous estimates of psychiatric morbidity for private households: about 1 in 7 adults (aged 16-64 years) had a diagnosable neurotic disorder in the week before interview, including mixed anxiety and depressive disorder (7.7%) and generalised anxiety disorder (3.1%), compared with 0.4% with a functional psychosis (schizophrenia or severe affective disorder) in a survey during 1993. Further reports are expected in 1995.

The Public Information Strategy on mental health published further booklets on mental health and older people[18], children and adolescents[19] and *What you can do about it*[20]; and a Focus on World Mental Health Day stimulated many local initiatives. A repeat of the attitudes to mental illness survey done in 1993 confirmed that the general population agrees with statements sympathetic to people with mental illness, but does still stigmatise them to some extent (DH Public Attitudes Survey, unpublished data). Pilot studies of the Health of the Nation outcome scales (HoNOS) to measure the health and social functioning of mentally ill people have been successfully completed and training packages are being developed[21].

Developments to improve purchasing of mental health services included initiatives from the Mental Health Task Force and the establishment of a branch of the NHS Executive with a specific responsibility to implement mental health policy. A London project was set up to visit all purchasing authorities, providers of health care and social services departments, and to develop action plans to address the concerns about bed pressures and the development of community services; a repeat visit to each authority at the end of the year reviewed progress. A second edition of the key area handbook was published including further information on bed management, targeting services and the care programme approach[22].

Discussion and debate on suicide prevention focused the attention of mental health teams, GPs and members of the public on various key issues and guidance, which included information on risk assessment, was disseminated[23]. Occupational groups at higher than usual risk of suicide among their members continued to develop strategies to help their peers through provision of helplines and other measures. The Medical Research Council (MRC) agreed to fund research specifically into suicide.

The Confidential Inquiry into Homicides and Suicides published a preliminary report into homicides[24] (see page 142).

(iv)   HIV/AIDS and sexual health

The Health of the Nation objectives for HIV/AIDS and sexual health are to reduce the incidence of HIV infection and other sexually transmitted diseases (STDs) and to reduce unwanted pregnancies[8]. £8 million were allocated to the HEA, £1.5 million to run the National AIDS Helpline and £49 million to the NHS for all forms of prevention activities. About half the NHS allocation is spent on public education, and half on protecting the blood supply, providing testing facilities, and staff training. HIV/AIDS is described in more detail in Chapter 6.

A related Health of the Nation target is to reduce the percentage of injecting drug misusers who report sharing injection equipment in the previous four weeks from 20% in 1990 to no more than 10% by 1997, and no more than 5% by the year 2000. Nationally, the percentage of notified drug misusers who inject drugs rose slightly from 54% to 56% in 1993, after successive annual falls from 67% in 1989. The most significant increase in injecting was among new addicts aged between 21 and 25 years, which rose from 56% in 1992 to 61% in 1993[25]. A small survey of 189 drug misusers in East Anglia during 1994 revealed that 12% had shared injecting equipment in the past four weeks; this was a significant drop from the 21% who reported sharing in a similar survey in 1993[26]. A report will be commissioned to advise on further monitoring of this equipment-sharing target, including those drug misusers not in touch with health services.

The number of new cases of gonorrhoea seen at NHS genito-urinary medicine (GUM) clinics continued to fall in 1993 (down 17% compared with 1992). The incidence of new cases per 100,000 population aged 15-64 years fell to 38; the Health of the Nation target to reduce this incidence to no more than 49 per 100,000 by 1995 has already been met.

In 1991, the conception rate among girls aged under 16 years fell for the first time in ten years, by approaching 10% compared with 1990. In 1992, the rate fell by nearly 10% to 8.4 per 1,000. The teenage abortion rate fell from 17.3 per 1,000 in 1992 to 16.5 in 1993. NHS priorities guidance for 1995/96[27] requires health authorities to achieve further improvements in this key area.

In March, DH funded two publicity campaigns to promote progress on prevention of unwanted pregnancy. The first, developed by the Family Planning Association, used radio advertisements to get parents to talk to their children about sex and contraception and offered a free booklet *Answering your child's questions*[28]. The other, 'Sexwise', offered young people a free, confidential phoneline and the opportunity to talk to a trained advisor about sex and personal relationships. Both campaigns were successful and research into the 'Sexwise' campaign indicated considerable demand for an anonymous, confidential telephone service.

(v)   Accidents

The Health of the Nation White Paper[8] set clear targets to reduce death rates from accidents by 33% among children aged under 15 years by 2005 (compared with a 1990 baseline). For young people aged 15-24 years the reduction target was 25%, and for elderly people (aged over 65 years), 33%. For a typical NHS Trust serving a population of 250,000, this would mean an overall reduction in deaths from accidents of: one among children aged under 15 years; two among young people aged 15-24 years; and five among people aged 65 years and over.

Encouraging progress seems to have been made towards the achievement of these targets among children and young adults, but deaths among the elderly rose[29]. Some of this rise among elderly people may be accounted for by the increasing numbers of very elderly people (aged over 85 years). These data will be closely monitored.

The Accident Prevention Task Force, set up in 1992 - which includes representatives of eight Government Departments, local authorities, voluntary organisations, the police, schools and universities, nursing and industry - has continued to emphasise the need to identify the causes of and risk factors for accidents, and to evaluate effective programmes of intervention to prevent accidents. During 1994, a review of published research was commissioned from the London School of Hygiene and Tropical Medicine. This report provides an overview of research published on the three age-groups targeted in the Health of the Nation[30], and notes uneven standards - such as poor research design with insufficient attention to evaluation; a lack of standard definitions (eg, in describing a fall or serious injury); a lack of information on cost and cost-effectiveness of interventions; and a lack of multidisciplinary research on risk avoidance that might be generally applicable to accident prevention. The Task Force agreed to obtain information on research planned and in progress via questionnaires sent to 100 organisations concerned with accident prevention, and will use the returns to compile a research strategy which can be made available to commissioners and funders of research, as well as to researchers.

A report by DH's Public Health Information Strategy team in 1993 described and assessed the potential of existing accident data collection systems[31]. Work continued in 1994 to identify changes that will be required to improve linkage and the means by which the information on the causes, severity and outcome of accidental injuries treated in NHS accident and emergency departments might be extended. Arrangements were also made to include incidence of accidental injuries in a population-based health survey to be carried out in England during 1995, which will measure numbers, severity and causes of unreported injuries and identify the toll that accidents take on health in comparison with disease.

References

1. Sharp I, ed. *Coronary heart disease: are women special?*. London: National Forum for Coronary Heart Disease Prevention, 1994.
2. Pettigrew M, McKee M, Jones J. Coronary artery surgery: are women discriminated against? *BMJ* 1993; **306**: 1164-6.
3. Clarke KW, Gray D, Keating NA, Hampton JR. Do women with acute myocardial infarction receive the same treatment as men? *BMJ* 1994; **309**: 563-6.
4. Nursing Times. *Women's health: a Nursing Times special review*. London: Macmillan Magazines, 1994.
5. Office of Population Censuses and Surveys. *Health Survey for England 1992*. London: HMSO, 1994.
6. Department of Health, Central Health Monitoring Unit. *Coronary heart disease: an epidemiological overview*. London: Department of Health, 1994.
7. Department of Health, Central Health Monitoring Unit. *Stroke: an epidemiological overview*. London: Department of Health, 1994.
8. Department of Health. *The Health of the Nation: a strategy for health in England*. London: HMSO, 1992 (Cm. 1986).
9. Department of Health. *Cervical cytology 1993/94. Summary information from Form KC53, England*. London: Department of Health (in press).

10. Anglia and Oxford Regional Health Authority, NHS Cervical Screening Programme National Co-ordinating Network. *Assuring the quality and measuring the effectiveness of cervical screening.* Oxford: Anglia and Oxford Regional Health Authority, 1994.
11. Anglia and Oxford Regional Health Authority, NHS Cervical Screening Programme National Co-ordinating Network. *Report of the first five years of the NHS cervical screening programme.* Oxford: Anglia and Oxford Regional Health Authority, 1994.
12. Department of Health. *On the State of the Public Health: the annual report of the Chief Medical Officer of the Department of Health for the year 1993.* London: HMSO, 1994; 63.
13. Melia J, Bulman A. Sunburn and tanning in a British population. *J Publ Health Med* (in press).
14. Office of the Population Censuses and Surveys. *Cancer statistics registrations: registrations of cancer diagnosed: England and Wales: 1989.* London: HMSO, 1994 (Series MB1 no. 22).
15. Standing Medical Advisory Committee. *Management of lung cancer: current clinical practices: report of a working group.* London: Department of Health, 1994. Chair: Professor Michael Whitehouse.
16. Department of Health. Management of lung cancer. *CMO's Update* 1994; **4:** 4, 8.
17. Meltzer H. *The prevalence of psychiatric morbidity among adults aged 16-64 living in private households in Great Britain.* London: OPCS, 1994 (OPCS Surveys of Psychiatric Morbidity in Great Britain; Bulletin 1).
18. Department of Health. *Mental illness: mental health and older people.* Heywood (Lancashire): Department of Health, 1994.
19. Department of Health. *Mental illness: can children and young people have mental health problems?* Heywood (Lancashire): Department of Health, 1994.
20. Department of Health. *Mental illness: what you can do about it.* Heywood (Lancashire): Department of Health, 1994.
21. Department of Health. HoNOS: a psychiatric thermometer. *CMO's Update* 1994; **4:** 7.
22. Department of Health. *The Health of the Nation Key Area Handbook: mental illness, 2nd edn.* London: Department of Health, 1994.
23. Jenkins R, Griffiths S, Wylie I, Hawton K, Morgan G, Tylee A. *The prevention of suicide.* London: HMSO, 1994.
24. Royal College of Psychiatrists. *A preliminary report on homicide.* London: Royal College of Psychiatrists, 1994.
25. Home Office. *Statistics of drug addicts notified to the Home Office: United Kingdom: 1993.* London: Home Office, 1994 (Statistical Bulletin: 10/94).
26. Anglia and Oxford Regional Health Authority. *Sharing injecting equipment: report of the survey in East Anglia in 1994.* Oxford: Anglia and Oxford Regional Health Authority, 1994.
27. Department of Health. *Priorities and planning guidance 1995/96.* Leeds: NHS Executive, 1994 (Executive Letter: EL(94)55).
28. Family Planning Association. *Answering your child's questions.* London: Family Planning Association, 1991.
29. Department of Health. *Public health common data set.* Guildford: University of Surrey, Institute of Public Health, 1993. (Data definitions and user guide for computer files; vol 1.)
30. Department of Health, London School of Hygiene and Tropical Medicine, Higginson I. *The Health of the Nation accident reduction targets: a research overview: what further research is needed?* Heywood (Lancashire): Department of Health (in press).
31. Department of Health. *Improving information on accidents.* Leeds: Department of Health, 1993 (Public Health Information Strategy; Implementation Project no. 19).

(c)   Implementation

(i)   Priorities for the NHS

The strategy for health[1] was again identified as a top objective for the NHS in 1994/95 and 1995/96 in its *Priorities and planning guidance*[2,3], ensuring that the key areas and other White Paper objectives remain at the top of the NHS management agenda.

At local level, Health of the Nation objectives continue to be reflected in corporate contracts, joint purchasing plans, service agreements and a great variety of initiatives by District Health Authorities (DHAs), hospital and community units, and primary health care teams. This work ensures that commitments made in Regional corporate contracts are underpinned by local management action and by suitable local programmes that cover health promotion and, where necessary, an increased focus on health outcomes in secondary care within the five key areas.

The Health of the Nation White Paper[1] identified the need for Regional Health Authorities (RHAs) to agree local targets which represent their contribution towards the national targets, but which also reflect additional local health priorities; these have been agreed. The NHS Executive is now working to improve the availability of management information, particularly at DHA level, to track progress in the implementation of the strategy.

The NHS Executive followed up the commitment in the White Paper to develop the concept of healthy hospitals by holding a series of consultative workshops in the Autumn of 1993. The resulting guidance document, *Health promoting hospitals*[4], was published in September 1994. The Executive also runs a central database and support unit to share best practice and to encourage a network of healthcare organisations in England committed to the Health of the Nation initiative.

The Chief Medical Officer issued a challenge during 1993 to every person in England to take steps to reduce personal risks of preventable illness and to improve their own health[5], which was successfully taken up by a wide range of organisations. Distribution of this challenge was continued in 1994 throughout the NHS and to individuals with an interest in it, such as patients and carers.

In July, the Chief Medical Officer asked Sir Christopher Paine, President of the Royal College of Radiologists, to chair a Working Party to improve hospital doctors' knowledge of the Health of the Nation initiative. Specific information for hospital doctors will be published in Spring 1995, and health promotion in postgraduate training and ways in which hospital doctors can contribute to the commissioning process have been reviewed.

DH funded a one-day conference in November to look at the implications of the results of the Oxcheck[6] and Family Heart[7] studies. The conference agreed that health promotion should be an essential part of primary care in the prevention of cardiovascular disease, but the amount of information collected should be reduced and more emphasis put on improving the quality of interventions. A report of the conference will be published during 1995. A multidisciplinary Mental Health Purchasing Workshop to improve purchasing of adult mental health services to complement those of primary care providers took place in February. The recommendations and examples of good practice are being taken forward. A primary care handbook[8] which described the role of all members of the wider primary care team in helping to improve the Health of the Nation was issued in September not only to GPs and associated practice staff, but also to pharmacists, dentists, optometrists and community nursing and dental staff.

Eat Well![9], the Nutrition Task Force (NTF) programme for meeting the Health of the Nation diet and nutrition targets, identified a range of priorities for co-ordinated action. Following publication of its programme in March, the NTF launched a nutrition handbook for NHS managers in June to help those involved in translating the targets into action[10]; a National Food Guide for educators and communicators in July[11]; and a core curriculum document on the nutrition education of health professionals in November[12], which aimed to help educational establishments as they adapt their curricula to reflect the Health of the Nation targets (see page 69).

(ii)   *Local health alliances*

The Health of the Nation initiative recognises as one of its key themes that health is not a matter simply for the NHS or for DH, but stresses the importance of alliances in which a number of partners come together for the shared purpose of improving health. To encourage such joint working, the Health Alliance Awards Scheme was launched in July to highlight examples of good practice.

This scheme will run at regional and national levels. At regional level, there are six awards - one for each of the key areas and one for alliances whose work spans two or more of them. Regional winners in each category will come forward to the national competition, which has an additional category for alliances whose work is nationwide. By the closing date in November, 320 entries had been received which showed an encouraging spread of partners. Many, though by no means all, involved the NHS; but there was also clear evidence of commitment from local authorities, voluntary bodies, universities and many other organisations in a wide variety of enterprising and innovative schemes. Judging will take place early in 1995.

(iii)   *Healthy settings*

The Health of the Nation White Paper[1] identified a range of 'healthy settings' in which activity towards achieving its targets could be given specific focus - cities, schools, hospitals, the workplace, homes, prisons, and the environment. The entire population is covered in one or more of these settings. During 1994, 16 pilot schools and 32 reference schools were chosen to participate in the European network of health promoting schools. In the Autumn, the NHS Executive produced a document to explain the concept of health promoting hospitals[4] and will continue to develop a network of participating hospitals and to maintain a database to help to share good practice. All prison establishments are now required to develop health promotional programmes. A Workplace Steering Group is developing a plan of action to encourage workplace health promotion, concentrating on the advantages of healthy alliances, and the NHS Executive has commissioned the HEA to take forward the 'Health at Work in the NHS' programme, with examples of good practice sent quarterly to all NHS work sites.

(iv)   Inter-Departmental co-operation

The Health of the Nation White Paper[1] was published as a Government document, not from the Department of Health alone. This distinction recognised that many Government Departments and Agencies have responsibility for areas of policy that have direct impact on the health of the population. Examination of the healthy settings initiative shows this range: for example, the Department for Education takes the lead in schools; the Home Office in prisons; the Department of the Environment in the environment, in cities and in homes; and the Department of Employment in the workplace. Within the key areas the Department of Transport has a strong interest in accidents and the Ministry of Agriculture, Fisheries and Food in nutrition targets for CHD and stroke. At local level, several of the entries for the Health Alliance Awards are part of the Department of the Environment's City Challenge initiative. Task Forces and Working Groups set up to promulgate the strategy for health often include representatives from several Government Departments and Agencies (such as the HEA and the Health and Safety Executive), as well as independent experts.

References

1. Department of Health. *The Health of the Nation: a strategy for health in England.* London: HMSO, 1992 (Cm. 1986).
2. Department of Health. *Priorities and planning guidance 1994/95.* Leeds: NHS Management Executive, 1993 (Executive Letter: EL(93)54).
3. Department of Health. *Priorities and planning guidance for the NHS 1995/96.* Leeds: NHS Executive, 1994 (Executive Letter: EL(94)55).
4. Department of Health. *Health promoting hospitals.* Heywood (Lancashire): Department of Health, 1994.
5. Department of Health. *Chief Medical Officer's Challenge.* Heywood (Lancashire): Department of Health, 1993.
6. Imperial Cancer Research Fund OXCHECK Study Group. Effectiveness of health checks conducted by nurses in primary care: results of the OXCHECK study after one year. *BMJ* 1994; **308:** 308-12.
7. Family Heart Study Group. Randomised controlled trial evaluating cardiovascular screening and intervention in general practice: principal results of British family heart study. *BMJ* 1994; **308:** 313-20.
8. Department of Health. *Health of the Nation: an introductory booklet for the primary care team.* Heywood (Lancashire): Department of Health, 1994.
9. Department of Health. *Eat well! An action plan from the Nutrition Task Force to achieve the 'Health of the Nation' targets on diet and nutrition.* Heywood (Lancashire): Department of Health, 1994. Chair: Professor Dame Barbara Clayton.
10. Department of Health. *Nutrition and health: a management handbook for the NHS.* Heywood (Lancashire): Department of Health, 1994.
11. Health Education Authority. *The national food guide: the balance of good health.* London: Health Education Authority, 1994.
12. Department of Health. *Nutrition: core curriculum for nutrition in the education of health professionals.* London: Department of Health, 1994.

(d)   The way ahead

A strategy such as the Health of the Nation initiative cannot simply stay still. Indeed, the White Paper[1] explicitly stated that it was not the last word on the subject, but the beginning of a continuing process. Movement towards the targets feeds into the strategy's continual development, with initiatives generated and varied to concentrate work where it is most needed. Present indications are that targets related to obesity, suicide (particularly in young men) and teenage smoking will require particular attention in the immediate future.

Many of the targets are timed for the year 2000. Steady progress is needed if these are to be reached and it will be important that the strategy does not lose its focus or momentum in the meantime. A key element will be the development of an effective communications strategy to raise the profile of the Health of the Nation further among purchasers and providers of care (including the NHS, local authorities and voluntary organisations); the media and other opinion formers; and the public at large.

A communications team was set up in October and is developing a series of themes to give fresh perspectives and pull together work across the five key areas - with special initiatives to target young people, people at work, and the elderly. The first of these, Health of the Young Nation, will pick up concerns about adolescent health set out in last year's Report[2], and provide a focus for the wider community to tackle health problems that affect or worry young people so as to improve the health of the future nation.

It is also essential to make better use of people outside Government to get messages across. Business partnerships spread health messages through outlets such as leisure centres and supermarkets, as well as in the workplace, and are developing a series of themed health challenges - the first three being sun, safety and food - to follow on from the Chief Medical Officer's challenge to the nation as a whole. The communications team will also build on health alliances between local authorities, community groups, voluntary organisations and schools, and co-ordinate action by producing a wall-chart, a compendium of events and other publications to help those working on the strategy for health in Government Departments, NHS Regions, the HEA and other organisations.

Better communication of Health of the Nation initiative within the NHS is also essential and the communications team is working closely with the NHS Executive and Regions to assess the gaps that need to be filled and the techniques that have proved to be effective, including the better use of information technology for education and mass communication. Finally, the communications team is exploring ways to make better use of video news releases, radio tapes, features in the specialist press, and more general media coverage to advance the goals of the Health of the Nation initiative.

References

1.   Department of Health. *The Health of the Nation: a strategy for health in England.* London: HMSO, 1992 (Cm. 1986).
2.   Department of Health. *On the State of the Public Health: the annual report of the Chief Medical Officer of the Department of Health for the year 1993.* London: HMSO, 1994; 5, 74-112.

CHAPTER 4

HEALTH IN THE WORKPLACE

(a)   Introduction

The first comprehensive text on occupational diseases was written by Professor Bernardino Ramazzini[1], a 17th Century Italian physician, who advised examining doctors to ask of patients: "What is your occupation?". Only in this way can the patient with work-related ill-health be managed appropriately, and any necessary preventive action considered to help to control risks in the workplace. The advice is as pertinent today and, rather than simply recording a job title which may be unrevealing or even misleading, practitioners should identify what their patients' work actually involves and any associated hazards.

The Industrial Revolution in Britain brought large-scale manufacture of iron, cotton and woollen cloth, glass and other goods, and deep-mining of coal. Working conditions were often extremely poor and health suffered greatly. The efforts of philanthropists helped to highlight the problems and social reforms brought improvements. Charles Thackrah, the founder of the Leeds medical school, wrote a classic text on the health effects of "the principal arts, trades and professions" in 1831[2]. He focused on preventive aspects, as well as the identification and management of work-related illness, and had a broad concept of occupational health which embraced health and social issues in the home and general community.

Sir Thomas Legge, the first Medical Inspector of Factories, observed after his appointment in 1898 that "All workmen should be told something of the danger of the material with which they come in contact and not be left to find it out for themselves - sometimes at the cost of their lives"[3]. Since then, political will and economic progress have led to a well-developed regulatory system for health and safety at work[4], and enormous strides have been made in the prevention of serious and disabling disease and injury. While some of the traditional hazards still remain in certain types of work, and need continued vigilance, many of the classic industrial diseases, such as silicosis and heavy-metal poisoning, are becoming rarer due to better control of risks. However, other problems have assumed greater importance; new challenges have emerged, frequently multi-factorial and complex to control.

The amount of harm caused by accidents and health risks in the workplace is notoriously difficult to quantify. Despite the advances which have occurred, recent studies highlight a national burden of ill-health and injury which cannot be ignored. Results of the 1990 Labour Force Survey (LFS)[5] of a representative sample of the England and Wales population estimated 1.6 million accidents at work in the previous 12 months and 2.2 million cases of work-related illness[6]. In consequence, 30 million work days were lost and over 20,000 people forced to give up work. Although the LFS data are based on self-reported illness and injury, and may over-estimate work as the cause, this nevertheless represents a considerable amount of human suffering to workers and their families, and a heavy economic cost to the country. It has been estimated that the overall cost of work-related ill-health and accidents (including those which do not give rise to injury but are preventable by better management of safety) is between £11 billion and £16 billion every year - or 2-3% of gross domestic product[6].

References

1. Ramazzini B. *De Morbus Artificum Diatriba 1713*. In: Raffle PAB, Adams PH, Baxter PJ, Lee WR, eds. *Hunter's diseases of occupations, 8th edn*. London: Edward Arnold, 1994.
2. Thackrah CT. *The effects of the principal arts, trades and professions and the civic states and habits of living on health and longevity with particular reference to the trades and manufactures of Leeds; and suggestions for the removal of many of the agents which produce disease, and shorten the duration of life*. London: Longman, Rees, Orne, Brown and Green, 1831.
3. Kipling MA. *A brief history of HM Medical Inspectorate*. London: Health and Safety Executive, 1979.
4. Carter JT. In: Raffle PAB, Adams PH, Baxter PJ, Lee WR, eds. *Hunter's diseases of occupations, 8th edn*. London: Edward Arnold, 1994.
5. Office of Population Censuses and Surveys. *Labour Force Survey 1990*. London: HMSO, 1993.
6. Health and Safety Executive. *The costs to the British economy of work accidents and work-related ill health*. London: Health and Safety Executive, 1994.

(b)   Occupational health today

(i)   *The changing industrial base and pattern of employment*

In recent years there has been considerable change in the structure of employment:

-       part-time work and self-employment have increased sharply as a proportion of total employment;

-       females have increased from 38% to 44% of the labour force over the past twenty years; *and*

-       small businesses have become more important. Between 1987 and 1991 the share of total employment in workplaces with less than 25 employees increased from 28.5% to 31.1%.

The service sector now accounts for over 70% of employment, while manufacturing industries' share has fallen to below one-fifth. The occupational structure of employment has shifted toward non-manual work, particularly managerial and professional, and away from traditional manual jobs such as machine operation. These trends are likely to continue in the coming years, although at a reduced rate.

Some of these changes, such as the shift away from primary and manufacturing industry, have considerable implications for occupational health - although reductions in illnesses associated with declining heavy industries occur slowly due to long latency periods for diseases such as pneumoconioses. Other changes, such as the shift to non-manual jobs and new technology, are highlighting new or previously neglected forms of ill-health.

(ii)   Societal changes and public expectations

Workers have a right to a safe and healthy working environment. The perception and acceptance of risks by individuals and society depend upon a number of factors and vary over time. Pressure groups, often set up by sufferers from particular diseases, push for better compensation payments or seek action to tighten controls or to have them enforced more rigorously. Increasing attention is also being paid to prevention of diseases previously accepted as an inevitable consequence of work, such as musculo-skeletal disorders. However, some workers may be reluctant to complain or to report early symptoms of ill-health if they fear redundancy or other repercussions.

(iii)   International influences

A number of new European Community (EC) Directives came into effect in the early 1990s. These included a Framework Directive which gave employers a number of new general duties with an impact on occupational health. This Directive has been implemented in the UK by the Management of Health and Safety at Work Regulations 1992[1].

The current programme of the EC to the year 2000 has a greater focus on information, training and guidance on good practice, but discussions are under way or planned on a number of health-related subjects including physical agents (such as noise and vibration), health surveillance, occupational health services and stress.

The World Health Organization's (WHO's) policy for Europe includes reference to the health of people at work and aims for reductions in work-related diseases and injuries and implementation of health promotion activities[2].

References

1. *Management of Health and Safety at Work Regulations 1992*. London: HMSO, 1992.
2. World Health Organization. *'Health for All' targets: the health policy for Europe: updated edn.* Copenhagen: WHO, 1993.

(c)   What is occupational health?

Occupational health is concerned with protecting and maintaining the health of people at work. It has three main components: the first two - the effects of work on health and the effects of health on the capacity to work - are concerned with the employer's statutory duties to ensure employees' health and safety in the workplace; the third component - health promotion - is concerned with voluntary activities by the employer to educate and encourage workers to adopt healthier lifestyles. Knowledge of the working environment is vital to the effective practice of occupational health.

(i)   The effect of work on health

Almost half the population is employed and work is an important factor in people's health. However, about one in 14 family doctor consultations of people of working age involves work-related illness[1]. In 1990, 750,000 people took time off work for work-related ill-health and another 730,000 were affected by work-related illness but did not take time off because of it[1,2].

While some traditional occupational diseases like pneumoconioses and poisoning from heavy metals have declined, others such as dermatitis, deafness, musculo-skeletal disorders and asthma remain common and can be disabling. Acute or chronic harm from exposure to chemicals, biological agents or physical hazards at work can lead to serious illness or death where control measures are inadequate.

The causes of illness in the workplace can be hard to identify, but the key to prevention lies in early identification of problems and knowing what steps to take to reduce risks. Appropriate action by employers based on a thorough and well-informed assessment of risks can successfully tackle many hazards before anyone's health is affected. However, health surveillance and early diagnosis of illness which may be related to occupation provides another line of defence and an opportunity to take remedial action.

(ii)   The effect of health on work

Health assessments for fitness to work are designed to ensure that individuals are physically and mentally fit to perform relevant tasks effectively and without risk to themselves or their colleagues. When considering the employability of any individual, and particularly those with health problems or disabilities, the occupational health practitioner needs to know and to understand the environment in which they work and the range of duties to be performed. Thus an assessment can be made of the mental and physical capacity of the individual for the tasks involved. As well as considering ability to carry out the work, health and safety implications require careful appraisal in terms of any risks to the individual or to others[3].

(iii) Health promotion

In the UK, almost half the population is employed (or self-employed) and many individuals spend about half their waking hours at work on working days. This provides relative ease of access for health promotion on a regular basis to large numbers of people, including younger age-groups who might not otherwise benefit from direct health-promoting activity. Policies can be formulated on 'healthy lifestyle' issues such as discouraging smoking, and encouraging healthier eating, sensible drinking and physical exercise. The potential benefits are considerable: smoking is the largest preventable cause of death[4], and alcohol and smoking together account for 60 million lost working days annually.

Nevertheless, careful attention needs to be given to the likely benefits and cost-effectiveness of interventions. Health promotion programmes should have clear aims and objectives, and measurable outcomes; as in other areas of practice, activity should be audited. It is important to secure the commitment of senior management and employees alike, and to take account of the needs of the particular business in designing a programme.

References

1. McCormick A, Fleming D, Charlton J. *Morbidity Statistics from General Practice: fourth national study: 1991-92.* London: HMSO (in press).
2. Office of Population Censuses and Surveys. *General Household Survey 1993.* London: HMSO (in press).
3. Cox RAF, Edwards FC, McCallum RI, eds. *Fitness for work: the medical aspects, 2nd edn.* Oxford: Oxford University Press (in press).
4. Department of Health, Health Education Authority. *Creating effective smoking policies in the NHS.* London: Health Education Authority, 1992.

(d)   Legislative and organisational framework

The law on occupational health

The Health and Safety at Work etc. Act 1974[1] places general duties on all people at work. It was superimposed on earlier legislation, parts of which remain in force, but an objective of the Act is gradually to replace old law with a modern system of regulation. Much progress has been made. A series of new regulations and approved codes of practice now sets out requirements in more detail than the Act; some apply to most or all workplaces, but many deal with special circumstances or particular hazards. Wherever possible, this modern legislation sets goals and avoids prescriptive detail.

The 1974 Act requires employers to ensure, so far as is reasonably practicable, the health, safety and welfare at work of their employees, and others who may be affected by their activities. Employees have a duty to take reasonable care for their own safety, and that of others. More recent regulations, such as the Management of Health and Safety at Work Regulations 1992[2] have added new general duties for employers to carry out risk assessments; to take appropriate preventive and protective measures; and to have access to competent help in applying health and safety law. A considerable amount of guidance on regulations has also been published.

Mechanisms for law and standard making

The 1974 Act[1] set up the Health and Safety Commission (HSC) and the HSE. The HSC is responsible to Ministers for promoting the objectives of the Act; it has a chairman and nine members, including representatives of employer, employee and local authority organisations. HSE acts for HSC in carrying out the work necessary for it to perform its functions, and has responsibility for enforcement of the law. Its field force comprises several Inspectorates and the Employment Medical Advisory Service[3]. Environmental health officers enforce health and safety law in lower-risk premises, such as shops and offices.

The fundamental aim of HSC and HSE is to ensure that risks to people's health and safety from work activities are properly controlled. They provide a framework of law and standards; promote new research on hazards and prevention; provide advice and guidance to employers, workers and the public; inspect workplaces; and, if persuasion fails, issue improvement or prohibition notices or prosecute under statutory provisions. The policy work of HSC is assisted by a network of expert industry advisory committees and subject advisory committees, including an occupational health advisory committee.

References

1. *Health and Safety at Work Act etc. 1974.* London: HMSO, 1994.
2. *Management of Health and Safety at Work Regulations 1992.* London: HMSO, 1992.
3. Carter JT. Twenty one years of EMAS. *Occup Med* 1994; **44:** 119-22.

(e)   Information about occupational ill-health

No single source of information about occupational illness can provide the full statistical picture. There are five main sources of information, with different characteristics in terms of coverage, completeness and reliability.

Under the Industrial Injuries Scheme, compensation may be payable for occupational diseases which appear on the list of prescribed diseases. The Industrial Injuries Advisory Council (IIAC) provides independent advice on the prescription of industrial diseases and on the Industrial Injuries Scheme. Diseases are only prescribed where the link with specific occupational causes is well established and certain qualifying conditions are met. There are 66 prescribed diseases, but approximately 75% of new assessments of disablement during 1991-92 were in respect of six diseases - occupational deafness, vibration white finger, diffuse mesothelioma, pneumoconiosis, occupational asthma, and tenosynovitis (see Tables 4.1 and 4.2). In future years the pattern will be influenced by claims for chronic bronchitis and emphysema, prescribed for underground coal miners and introduced in September 1993.

A second major source of information is the medical profession. In contrast to some other countries, there is no general legal requirement on doctors to report cases of disease with a suspected occupational cause. However, in two specialties where such causes are relatively common - dermatology and respiratory disease - voluntary reporting schemes have been set up. SWORD (surveillance of work-related and occupational respiratory disease) - a project run by the National Heart and Lung Institute in collaboration with the Society of Occupational Medicine, the British Thoracic Society and the HSE - has been in operation since 1989, and EPI-DERM (surveillance of skin diseases), has been run by the Centre for Occupational Health, University of Manchester, since 1993. Under these schemes, specialists in respiratory medicine, dermatology and occupational health make regular (quarterly for EPI-DERM, mostly monthly for SWORD) returns recording brief details of new cases of illness where they have established or suspect an occupational cause. Summaries of the accumulating

Table 4.1: *New cases of occupational lung diseases and deafness under the Industrial Injuries and Pneumoconiosis, Byssinosis and Miscellaneous Diseases Benefit Schemes, Great Britain, 1987-93*

Occupational lung disease/deafness	1987	1988	1989	1990	1991	1992	1993
Pneumoconiosis (except asbestosis)*	469	412	437	417	447	428	456
Asbestosis*	282	225	280	306	330	354	418
Byssinosis*	25	15	15	18	7	4	5
Farmers' lung	8	15	13	7	5	5	3
Occupational asthma	220	222	220	216	293	553	510
Mesothelioma	399	479	441	462	519	551	608
Lung cancer (asbestos)	55	59	54	58	55	54	72
Lung cancer (other prescribed agents)	0	0	4	6	6	6	3
Bilateral pleural thickening	115	114	125	146	149	160	172
Other occupational lung disease	10	5	0	4	6	5	2
Chronic bronchitis and/or emphysema†	..	..	..	..	..	..	1560
Occupational deafness	1202	1261	1170	1128	1041	972	901
All occupational lung diseases and deafness	2785	2807	2759	2768	2858	3092	4710

* Figures from 1990 do not include cases awarded by Medical Appeal Tribunals.
† Not applicable before 1993.

Source: DHSS/DSS

Table 4.2: *New cases of other occupational diseases under the Industrial Injuries Benefit Schemes, Great Britain, 1986-87 to 1992-93*

Other occupational diseases*	1986-87	1987-88	1988-89	1989-90	1990-91	1991-92	1992-93
Dermatitis	464	368	285	301	434	411	419
Tenosynovitis	376	322	294	423	556	649	911
Vibration white finger	1366	1673	1056	2601	5403	2369	1447
'Beat' conditions	57	171	112	95	187	317	456
Carpal tunnel syndrome†	..	..	..	..	..	..	20
Viral hepatitis	5	3	1	1	2	4	1
Tuberculosis	13	3	5	0	3	3	6
Leptospirosis	1	0	0	2	0	1	1
Other infections	5	0	1	2	5	4	3
Poisonings	9	2	16	6	4	8	9
Occupational cancers	27	29	11	18	17	23	30
Inflammation/ulceration of mucous membrane of upper respiratory tract	..	19	15	22	13	75	294
Other conditions	58	20	21	33	72	68	132
Total	*2381*	*2610*	*1817*	*3504*	*6696*	*3932*	*3729*

* From October 1986, disablement benefit was paid only for cases with disability assessed at 14% or more; the figures for 1986-87 and subsequent years include cases not qualifying for benefit but assessed at 1-13%; figures collected for years ending 30 September.
† Not applicable before 1992-93.

Source: DHSS/DSS

data are regularly reported back to the participating specialists. Fuller analyses are published in occupational medicine journals[1,2,3,4]. These sources provide additional information on the detail of presumed causative substances than is available from the Industrial Injuries Scheme, with wider coverage because cases are not required to fit precise prescription rules nor to cause long-term disablement. However, although participation rates in the relevant specialties are high (72% for SWORD, 67% for EPI-DERM), they are not complete.

An alternative view of occupational disease can be based on the opinions of those who are - or believe themselves to be - affected. In 1990, the HSE commissioned a supplementary series of questions in the Labour Force Survey[5]. All adults in a representative sample of 60,000 households in England and Wales were asked the question: "In the last 12 months, have you suffered from any illness, disability or other physical problem which was caused or made worse by your work. Please include any work you have done in the past". Those who responded positively were asked further questions about their illness and the job which they believed had caused or exacerbated it. They were also asked: "Was your illness caused by your work, or did your work simply make it worse?". Based on the response to this survey, work-related illness may affect about 6% of the adult population, with about half these cases 'caused' by work. Figure 4.1 shows the estimated prevalence of work-related illness by broad disease group. However, although such a population survey has the advantage of representative coverage of the whole population, it relies on the perceptions of the affected person.

The fourth major information source is provided by national mortality data. This can be used in two ways: a few occupational diseases - asbestosis, pneumonoconiosis, farmers' lung - have specific International Classification of Diseases (ICD) codes and can be monitored through routine national mortality statistics. The close association of mesothelioma with asbestos exposure, and the predominance of occupation as a source of asbestos exposure for individuals, means that although such deaths are not exclusively occupational, the trends in these deaths are an important indicator of occupational asbestos exposure. Finally, the analysis of cause-specific mortality data in relation to occupations recorded at death registration (the decedent's last full-time occupation) can indicate possible occupational health risks. Such analyses were pioneered in this country by Dr William Farr in a series of reports beginning in 1841, and have been published regularly as supplements to each decennial Census since 1861. The latest in the series will be published early in 1995[6].

The final source of ill-health information is the statutory system introduced by the Reporting of Injuries, Diseases and Dangerous Occurrences Regulations (RIDDOR) 1986[7]. These Regulations require employers to report all cases of a defined list of diseases occurring among their employees where:

-    they receive a doctor's written diagnosis; *and*

-    the affected employee's current job involves the work activity specifically associated with the disease.

Figure 4.1: *Estimated annual prevalence of self-reported work-related illness, by disease category, England and Wales, 1989/90*

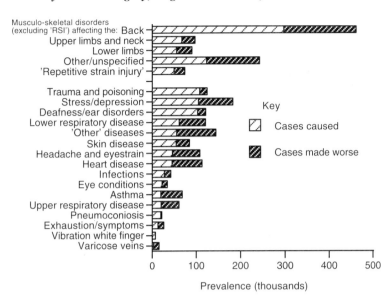

Note: Diseases ordered by number of cases 'caused', with musculo-skeletal conditions (including 'repetitive strain injury') treated as a group.

Source: OPCS, LFS

The list of diseases is similar to that in the Industrial Injuries Scheme but comparison with the scheme suggests substantial under-reporting under RIDDOR. In practice, the main use of RIDDOR disease reports is not to construct a statistically valid database, but to trigger a visit from an employment medical adviser so that the employer can be advised of the remedial action needed to prevent a recurrence.

References

1. Meredith SK. Reported incidence of occupational asthma in the UK 1989-90. *J Epidemiol Commun Health* 1993; **47:** 459-63.
2. Meredith SK, McDonald C. Work-related respiratory disease in the UK 1989-92: a report on the SWORD project. *Occup Med* 1994: **44:** 183-89.
3. Meredith SK, Taylor VM, McDonald JC. Occupational respiratory disease in the United Kingdom: 1989: a report to the British Thoracic Society and the Society of Occupational Medicine by the SWORD project group. *Br J Indust Med* 1991; **48:** 292-8.
4. Health and Safety Commission. *Health and safety statistics: statistical supplement to the 1993/94 annual report.* London: Health and Safety Executive, 1994.
5. Office of Population Censuses and Surveys. *Labour Force Survey 1990.* London: HMSO, 1993.
6. Office of Population Censuses and Surveys, Health and Safety Executive. *Occupational Health Decennial Supplement (Series DS no 10).* London, HMSO (in press).
7. *Reporting of Injuries, Diseases and Dangerous Occurrences Regulations (RIDDOR) 1986.* London: HMSO, 1986.

(f) Main occupational health hazards, diseases and disorders

The following descriptions do not provide a comprehensive list of all workplace hazards and occupational diseases, but provide a very brief overview of some important areas.

(i)   *Chemical risks and diseases*

Some 'traditional' occupational diseases such as byssinosis (from cotton dust) have fallen to a very low level, reflecting both improved working conditions and a general decline in the industry (see Figure 4.2). Pneumoconioses as a result of exposure to coal dust and silica is also falling, but more slowly[1]. Pneumoconioses have a long latency between exposure and onset of disease, and are rarely seen within 10 years from first exposure, and in most cases appear after 15 to 30 years: thus new cases largely reflect the working conditions of 10 or more years ago (see Table 4.3 and Figure 4.3).

Asbestos

Four diseases have been unequivocally linked to asbestos exposure - asbestosis, mesothelioma, lung cancer and pleural thickening. The number of deaths attributable to asbestos exposure has been steadily rising for the last 20 years (see Figures 4.4 and 4.5 and Table 4.3), and it is estimated that asbestos is currently responsible for 3,000-3,500 deaths annually. The number of mesothelioma deaths is expected to go on rising until the year 2010, and possibly up to the year 2025. Age-specific rates in successive birth cohorts show increasing rates from the end of the last century up to the early 1940s. Rates for more recent birth cohorts are lower. Assuming that the estimated ratio between cases of mesothelioma and asbestos-induced lung cancer remains unchanged, it is expected that there may eventually be a peak of between 5,000 and 10,000 asbestos-related deaths annually[2].

Because of the long latency period for asbestos-related diseases, the deaths now occurring and those expected to occur in the future reflect industrial conditions of the past. This latency period means that the effectiveness of current regulations has yet to be demonstrated.

Other chemical carcinogens

A clear occupational link has been established for a relatively small percentage of cancers, in addition to asbestos-related lung cancer and mesothelioma. This has been possible for workplace exposure to a known carcinogen or where an association has been shown, for example, between occurrence of a rare cancer and work in a specific industry or job. Cancer of the nose and nasal sinuses has been associated with hardwood dust, with a relative risk for cabinet-makers of eight times that of the general population. Similarly, a link has been established between exposure to aromatic amines in the rubber industry and bladder cancer, nickel and nasal and lung cancer, vinyl chloride and angiosarcoma of the liver, and mineral oils and skin cancer, to name a few[3].

It has been estimated that around 4% (with a range of 2-8%) of all cases of cancer[4] could be avoided by the elimination of all workplace carcinogenic risks, including asbestos exposure - equivalent to some 6,000 premature deaths

Figure 4.2: *Disablement benefits and deaths attributed to byssinosis, Great Britain, 1973-93*

Number of cases

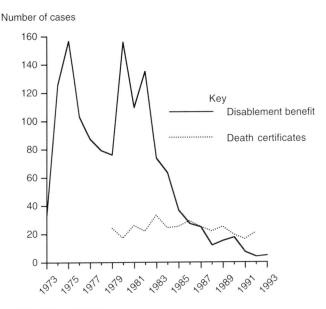

Source: DHSS/DSS and OPCS

Figure 4.3: *Disablement benefits (by coal and other sectors), death benefits and death certificates attributed to pneumoconioses (excluding asbestosis), Great Britain, 1971-93*

Number of cases

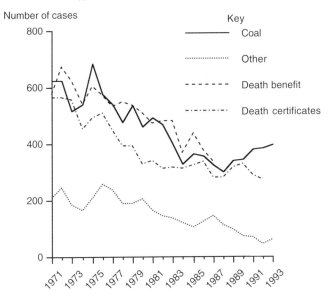

Note: From 1990, disablement figures do not include cases awarded by Medical Appeals Tribunals

Source: DHSS/DSS and OPCS

Table 4.3: *Deaths due to occupationally related lung disease, Great Britain, 1981-92*

Disease	1981	1982	1983	1984	1985	1986	1987	1988	1989	1990	1991	1992
Mesothelioma*	468	502	569	618	614	700	808	862	899	880	1009	..
Asbestosis excluding mesothelioma*	137	128	121	129	140	166	144	152	157	164	163	..
Pneumoconiosis (other than asbestos)†	341	314	317	314	324	337	279	281	318	328	287	274
Byssinosis†	26	22	33	24	25	29	25	22	25	19	16	21
Farmers' lung and other occupational allergic alveolitis†	13	15	15	10	7	15	16	9	8	6	8	4
Total	*985*	*981*	*1055*	*1095*	*1110*	*1247*	*1272*	*1326*	*1407*	*1397*	*1483*	*299*

*Numbers of deaths with mesothelioma or asbestosis mentioned in any part of the death certificate; 1992 figures not available.

†Numbers of death certificates coded to one of these diseases as the underlying cause of death.

Source: OPCS

Figure 4.4: *Death benefits, death certificates and disablement benefits attributed to asbestosis, Great Britain, 1971-93*

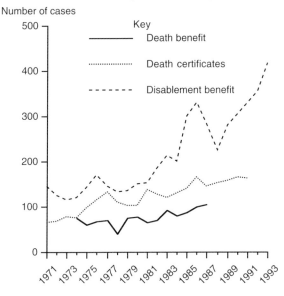

Note: From 1990 disablement benefit figures do not include cases awarded by Medical Appeals Tribunals

Source: DHSS/DSS and OPCS

Figure 4.5: *Death benefits, death certificates and disablement benefits attributed to mesothelioma, Great Britain, 1971-93*

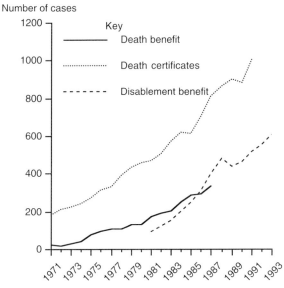

Note: 1987 is last full year for death benefit.
Disablement benefit figures not available for years to 1980.

Source: DHSS/DSS and OPCS

Table 4.4: *Estimated new cases of work-related and occupational respiratory disease, United Kingdom, 1993*

Disease	Number of cases
Allergic alveolitis	115
Asthma	912
Bronchitis	60
Building-related illness	23
Byssinosis	6
Infectious diseases	51
Inhalation accidents	295
Lung cancer	63
Malignant mesothelioma	700
Pleural disease (benign)	766
Pneumoconioses	385
Other	80
Total	*3456*

Source: SWORD

annually from work-related cancer. There is a need for better understanding of the relation between in-vitro and animal tests of carcinogenicity and human health risks. Astute clinical observation may lead to the suspicion of an occupational cancer, particularly one occurring earlier in life than would normally be expected. Occupational and environmental health surveillance through epidemiological methodologies may also highlight hitherto unsuspected associations or causal links between cancers and specific exposures or types of work.

Asthma and dermatitis are the major causes of ill-health as a result of current exposure to chemicals in the workplace. However, there is still a legacy of harm from past exposures to asbestos, coal dust and silica.

Occupational asthma

The LFS[5] estimates that 20,000 people believe that they have asthma caused by work and a further 50,000 believe their asthma is made worse by work. The SWORD scheme[6] recorded 912 new cases of occupational asthma in 1993, a slight fall from the previous year (see Table 4.4). Most people who develop occupational asthma do so in the first few months of exposure to the allergen, although sensitisation can occur after years of symptom-free exposure[7]. Thus occupational asthma is probably the major cause of respiratory ill-health in the UK resulting from today's working conditions. For some people with occupational asthma, the disease may persist long after exposure to the causative agent has stopped[8]. A better understanding of dose-response relations is emerging[9,10].

The SWORD scheme shows that over half the cases arise from just six main groups of agents (Figure 4.6). The main occupational groups affected are shown in Table 4.5. Coach and spray painters have by far the highest risk (658 cases

Figure 4.6: *Percentage incidence of occupational asthma by causative agent, United Kingdom, 1989*

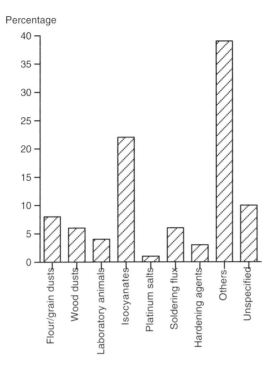

Source: SWORD

Table 4.5: *Substances responsible for most cases of occupational asthma*

Substance group	Examples of substances	Common activities
Isocyanates	TDI, MDI, HDI	Coach and other spray painting; foam manufacturing
Flour/grain/hay	Flour, barley, wheat oats, maize, rye	Handling grain at docks; milling, malting, baking
Soldering flux	Colophony fume	Welding, soldering, electronic assembly
Laboratory animals	Urine/dander from laboratory animals	Laboratory animal work
Wood dusts	African teak (iroko), western red cedar	Sawmilling, woodworking
Glues/resins	PA, TCPA, TMA, MA, MTPA	Curing of epoxy resins

TDI = toluene-2,4-di-isocyanate; MDI = diphenylmethane-di-isocyanate; HDI = hexamethylene-di-isocyanate; PA = phthalic anhydride; TCPA = tetrachlorophthalic anhydride; TMA = trimellitic anhydride; MA = maleic anhydride; MTPA = methyltetrahydrophthalic anhydride.

Source: SWORD

Table 4.6: *Reports of occupational asthma by occupational group and sex, United Kingdom, 1993*

Occupational group	Women Rate/million/ year	Men Rate/million/ year	All Rate/million/ year	95% CI
Professional, clerical and service work				
Laboratory technicians and assistants	203	174	188	139, 247
Cleaners	9	13	10	5, 16
Nurses	17	0	16	10, 24
Farmers and farm workers	43	24	28	18, 41
Hairdressers	87	0	81	46, 131
Remainder	3	3	3	2, 4
Material processors (excluding metal and electrical)				
Wood workers	35	54	54	40, 70
Food processors (excluding bakers)	146	90	108	75, 150
Bakers	364	314	334	248, 440
Plastics workers	163	386	337	248, 448
Chemical processors	271	377	364	274, 475
Remainder	41	53	49	39, 60
Metal and electrical processing and making				
Welding, soldering and electronic assembly	268	120	175	138, 218
Metal treatment	174	275	267	194, 360
Remainder	48	28	29	24, 35
Painting, assembly and packing				
Painters (excluding spray painters)	510	58	66	44, 95
Coach and other spray painters	450	663	658	508, 839
Remainder	31	41	36	26, 49
Construction and mining	64	11	11	7, 17
Transport and storage	0	8	8	5, 11

CI = Confidence interval.

Source: SWORD

per million exposed) as a result of spraying with paints that contain isocyanates (see Table 4.6). To reduce the incidence of the disease, HSE launched last April a 'Breathe Freely' campaign to raise awareness, particularly among small and medium-sized enterprises; it highlighted which substances cause occupational asthma and reminded employers of their duties to prevent or adequately to control exposure.

Data from the latest available year for SWORD are shown in Table 4.4. The category for allergic alveolitis includes cases of farmers' lung, mushroom-pickers' disease and similar conditions due to allergic reaction to fungal spores, moulds and other organic agents - conditions which can be disabling. Many cases are preventable if the necessary actions are taken in the workplace.

Dermatitis

The risk of dermatitis caused by an allergic or irritant reaction to substances used or handled at work applies to a wide range of jobs. The LFS[5] indicated that the numbers of people with skin disease caused or made worse by work were 54,000 and 30,000, respectively; over 90% of the cases reported arose as a result of a recent job (within the previous three years), suggesting that the condition is not persistent. Table 4.7 shows the agents most frequently reported to cause contact dermatitis in the EPI-DERM surveillance scheme[11]. Table 4.8 gives rates for the main occupational groups using information from EPI-DERM and numbers in each occupational group as projected by the LFS[5].

Other skin disorders are reported less commonly, including skin cancers, urticaria, trauma and infections.

Table 4.7: *Suspected agents most frequently reported for cases of contact dermatitis, United Kingdom, February 1993-April 1994*

Suspected agent	Males	Suspected agent	Females
Petroleum oils	141 *(11.8%)*	Nickel	240 *(23.3%)*
Rubber	132 *(11.0%)*	Unspecified irritants	148 *(14.4%)*
Unspecified irritants	117 *(9.8%)*	Wet work	146 *(14.2%)*
Chrome and chrome compounds	101 *(8.4%)*	Hairdressing chemicals	128 *(12.4%)*
Cutting oils	61 *(5.1%)*	Rubber	122 *(11.9%)*
All agents	1196 *(100%)*	All agents	1029 *(100%)*

Source: EPI-DERM

Table 4.8: *Rates of contact dermatitis by occupation, United Kingdom, February 1993-April 1994*

Recorded occupation	Rate (per 10,000)
Other labourers in making and processing industries	32.6
Hairdressers	16.7
Beauticians	8.6
Machine tool operatives	8.3
Printers	8.2
Chemical plant operatives	5.7
Labourers in engineering	5.5
Chefs and cooks	5.1
Paper, wood, plant operatives	5.1
Dental nurses	5.0
All occupations	*0.9*

Source: Cases reported to EPI-DERM compared with numbers in the Labour Force Survey[5].

Acute poisoning

A study commissioned by HSE of cases of poisoning by industrial chemicals in 1985 based on a 10% sample of attendances at NHS accident and emergency departments showed that 6% of attendances for ill-health related to toxic substances arose from work exposures[12]. This implies around 14,000 cases per year nationally - substantially more than the numbers reported under RIDDOR. Acids, alkalis, irritant vapours and solvents featured most commonly. Poisoning from gases, including carbon monoxide, comprises one-quarter of cases reported under RIDDOR.

Pesticide poisoning incidents are recorded in a 'green card' scheme operated by the West Midlands Poisons Unit in Birmingham. An estimated 70 poisoning cases per year ('confirmed' or 'likely') are due to pesticide exposure, most of which are relatively minor conditions. Many instances of ill-health related to pesticides affect members of the public, through indirect exposure, rather than workers handling substances directly.

(ii)   Physical risks and diseases

Musculo-skeletal risks and disorders

These form the largest single category of work-related illnesses in Britain by a wide margin. Latest estimates suggest an annual prevalence for musculo-skeletal disorders caused or made worse by work of 880,000, with about 5.5 million working days lost each year[5] (see Tables 4.9 and 4.10).

Work-related upper limb disorders is the preferred term to describe a range of disorders of the hand, wrist, arm, shoulder and neck, some of which are less accurately termed 'repetitive strain injury' (RSI). These disorders include medically well recognised ones - such as carpal tunnel syndrome, tenosynovitis and epicondylitis - as well as other more diffuse conditions such as shoulder girdle problems, the validity of which may be disputed. Various work and leisure factors can contribute to upper limb disorders, including awkward or static posture, excessive force, repetitive tasks, insufficient job rotation or psychological concerns. Work-related upper limb disorders occur in most industries, but the occupations at greatest risk include food processing, packaging, inspection and repetitive assembly work. Preventive solutions lie in the application of ergonomic principles to machinery design, layout of work-stations and task performance, and in organisational factors.

Manual handling - that is any movement of loads by use of human force - carries a risk of injury in many sectors of industry, but particularly in manufacturing and heavy industries such as mining and construction and in the armed forces. About 60,000 injuries reported to HSE and local authorities each year are caused or triggered by manual handling, which is approximately one-third of all reported injuries[12], ranging in severity from minor cuts, sprains and strains to permanent disablement; about half involve the back (see Figure 4.7). They are usually seen as acute incidents, but many are the result of cumulative injury and the longer-term effects of poor handling.

Special efforts have been made to tackle the problems of musculo-skeletal disorders. HSE has published extensive practical guidance for employers and employees and, over the past four years, has run a 'Lighten the Load' publicity and inspection campaign.

Hand-arm and whole-body vibration

Regular use of hand-held vibrating tools, such as road drills and chainsaws, can cause damage to the arteries, nerves, bones and muscles leading to a potentially disabling condition, hand-arm vibration syndrome (HAVS). The most common disorder is vibration white finger - periodic tingling, numbness and blanching of the fingers from impairment of blood-flow to them; painful throbbing may occur as blood returns after an attack. The 1990 Labour Force Survey[5] indicated a prevalence of 7,300 self-reported cases of vibration white finger, but other surveys suggest a higher estimate of around 20,000 cases[13]. The number of claimed cases for compensation under the Industrial Injuries Scheme has declined recently after a steady rise from 1985, when it was first prescribed (see Figure 4.8). However, in 1992-93 it was still the commonest prescribed disease, with 1,447 new cases awarded.

Little is known about the extent of whole-body vibration at work; it has been associated with back pain and other disorders. Unpublished HSE estimates indicate that up to 1.5 million workers could be at risk from low-back pain and other disorders from whole-body vibration, mainly from driving tractors and operating various types of machinery.

Table 4.9: *Estimated prevalence of self-reported work-related upper limb disorders, England and Wales, 1990*

Upper limb disorder	Prevalence	
	Total cases (thousands)	Cases felt to be caused by work (thousands)
Tenosynovitis	24.8	21.1
Bursitis	1.0	0.5
'RSI'	6.3	5.3
Tennis elbow	23.3	14.6
Carpal tunnel syndrome	4.2	2.3
Frozen shoulder	6.1	3.7
Non-specific musculo-skeletal	51.5	37.6
Rheumatoid arthritis	1.5	1.5
Arthritis	13.2	9.6
Spondylosis	8.4	5.0
Ankylosing spondylitis	0.9	0.0
Spondylitis	3.9	3.1
Rheumatism	2.5	2.0
Ganglion	1.1	0.0
Disc problems	3.6	2.0
Other musculo-skeletal	0.5	0.5
Trapped nerve	2.5	1.4
All upper limb disorders	*155.2*	*110.2*

'RSI' = 'Repetitive strain injury'.

Source: HSE

Table 4.10: *Estimated prevalence of self-reported work-related back disorders, England and Wales, 1990*

Back disorder	Prevalence	
	Total cases (thousands)	Cases felt to be caused by work (thousands)
Non-specific musculo-skeletal	257.1	170.7
Rheumatoid arthritis	1.5	0.6
Arthritis	26.2	14.3
Osteoarthritis	5.5	2.8
Sciatica	40.0	23.9
Spondylosis	1.0	0.5
Ankylosing spondylitis	1.0	1.0
Spondylitis	0.4	0.4
Rheumatism	0.5	0.5
Disc problems	110.3	70.1
Other musculo-skeletal	10.4	3.5
Trapped nerve	14.4	10.5
All back disorders	*468.4*	*298.8*

Source: HSE

Figure 4.7: *Estimated annual prevalence of self-reported work-related musculo-skeletal conditions by site, England and Wales, 1990*

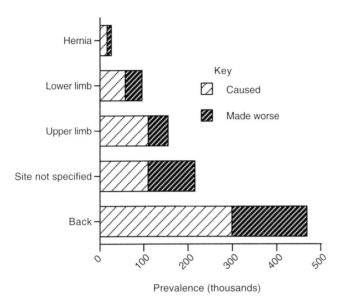

Prevalence (thousands)

Source: HSE

Figure 4.8: *New cases of vibration white finger diagnosed under Industrial Injuries Scheme, Great Britain, 1985-86 to 1992-93*

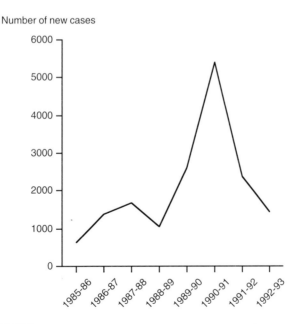

Source: DHSS/DSS

Noise

Prolonged exposure to high noise levels can result in noise-induced hearing loss (NIHL) and tinnitus. The decibel (dB) is the principal unit of sound pressure level, usually adjusted by an A-weighting to take account of the frequency response of human hearing. Its scale is logarithmic so that an increase of 3 dB(A) means a doubling of the sound power - typical noise levels are shown in Table 4.11. Regular exposure to noise levels above 85 dB(A) over an 8-hour working day is hazardous. Employers have a statutory duty to reduce noise levels as far as is reasonably practicable, and above 90 dB(A) they must provide workers with ear protection and ensure that it is worn[14]. Up to 1.5 million workers are exposed to hazardous noise, principally in construction, engineering, processing, mining and the armed forces. The OPCS Disability Surveys between 1985 and 1988 estimated that 52,500 people were affected by occupational deafness in England and Wales. The incidence rate of NIHL is now declining, partly as a result of the decline of heavy industry (see Figure 4.9).

Ionising radiation

Exposure to ionising radiation can occur in a wide range of occupations including the nuclear industry, the medical and dental professions, research laboratories and in some industrial processes. There are about 60,000 'classified' radiation workers (those who are likely to receive more than 30% of a relevant dose limit), while a further 100,000 are engaged in work in which they are exposed to a lesser dose. Exposure is typically from external photon radiation, with increased risk of developing cancers. Radiation doses to classified workers have fallen by more than half from 1986 to 1993 (see Figure 4.10), with a more than 10-fold decrease in the numbers who exceeded the regulatory investigation

Table 4.11: *Examples of typical noise levels and exposure times*

Noise level dB(A)	Noise source	Exposure time needed for daily dose of 90 dB(A)
0	Threshold of hearing	
20	Sound studio	
30	Quiet library	
40	Quiet office	
60	Conversation	
70	Loud radio	
80	Busy street	64 hours
90	Heavy lorry	8 hours
100	Pig house; weaving shed	50 minutes
115	Chainsaw; punch press	90 seconds
120	Riveting; boiler shop	30 seconds
138	Jet aircraft	< 1 second

Source: HSE

Figure 4.9: *New cases of occupational deafness diagnosed under Industrial Injuries Scheme, Great Britain, 1987-93*

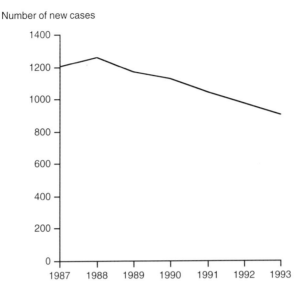

Number of new cases

Source: OPCS

level. The group with the highest average annual dose in 1992 was mining underground (non-coal), although industrial radiography on-site can also lead to high exposures.

Non-ionising radiation

Non-ionising radiation refers to photon emissions which do not have sufficient energy to ionise atoms; they include ultraviolet (UV), visible light, infra-red, microwave, radiofrequency and laser beams. UV radiation is a potential hazard for more than a million outdoor workers, and it can also be produced in a number of industrial activities, such as arc-welding. Exposure to electromagnetic fields (EMFs) at low intensities occurs in many occupations, but only high levels can produce adverse effects by increasing body temperature. Glass-workers and furnacemen are at risk of cataract from infra-red radiation[15]. A number of different health problems, including leukaemia, spontaneous miscarriage and altered mood, have allegedly been linked to EMFs[16], but evidence for a causal association is lacking. Working with visual display units has been queried as a possible cause of problems in pregnancy and harm to the unborn baby, but extensive scientific and medical analysis has failed to implicate EMFs as the cause[17].

In the case of environmental exposure to EMFs, living near overhead power lines has caused particular public health concern. Expert medical opinion does not confirm EMFs from such sources as a cause of cancer[18], but further work is in progress in response to recommendations that the possibility of an association be investigated further[19].

Figure 4.10: *Exposure to ionising radiation, all occupational categories, Great Britain, 1986-93*

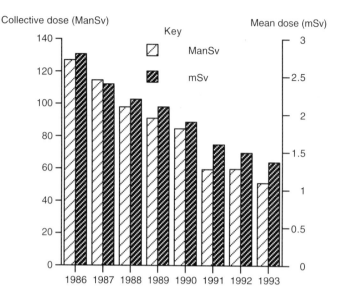

Source: HSE statistical summary from CIDI

Heat and cold

Thermal extremes can overcome the body's normal adaptive mechanisms and result in minor discomfort to severe distress and potentially death from heat stroke or hypothermia.

Work with compressed air

Caisson workers involved in tunnelling and underwater divers are exposed to hyperbaric pressures, and such workers require statutory medical examination by specially trained doctors approved by the HSE. Decompression sickness and other conditions are possible risks of this type of work.

(iii)   Biological hazards and diseases

Any definition of biological hazards needs to encompass all micro-organisms able to cause disease, and may also include reactions to plants and other living agents. In addition to illness from infection, micro-organisms can also have allergenic and toxic effects.

The 1990 LFS[5] indicated some 26,000 cases of ill-health as a result of infections thought to be related to work. However, this figure is likely to include many community-acquired infections. A number of initiatives are now being undertaken to establish a more systematic approach to the collection of data on ill-health due to exposure to biological hazards in the main occupational groups exposed, including a survey to investigate the incidence of work-related infection in the NHS.

The Advisory Committee on Dangerous Pathogens (ACDP), which is jointly serviced by DH and the HSE, advises the HSE, the HSC, and Ministers in DH and the Ministry of Agriculture, Fisheries and Food (MAFF) on all aspects of hazards and risks to workers and others from exposure to pathogens. The Committee produces guidance and advice on a range of issues, but particularly on worker safety.

The ACDP is preparing a report which will recommend principles for assessment of microbiological risks and, more specifically, its application to microbiological aspects of public health. ACDP publications on the categorisation of pathogens[20,21] set and help to maintain practical standards for the safe conduct of laboratory work with infectious agents. Both editions had the status of guidance supporting the Health and Safety at Work etc. Act 1974[22]. The Control of Substances Hazardous to Health (COSHH) Regulations 1988[23] and 1994[24] will be extended in 1995 to implement two EC Directives concerned with exposure to biological agents at work. Although still aimed primarily at workplaces where biological agents are handled intentionally (such as microbiology laboratories and in research and industry), a further edition of ACDP guidance, to be published in 1995, will be a useful source of information more generally.

Blood-borne infections

Blood-borne viruses present a potential hazard to workers at risk of exposure to blood, body fluids or blood-contaminated sharp objects. Employers are required to undertake appropriate risk assessments and to draw up and implement policies to protect such workers. Health care workers are at particular risk of exposure: in 1990, the UK Health Departments published guidance for clinical health care workers on protection against infection with HIV and hepatitis viruses[25].

The ACDP first published guidance on HIV and AIDS in 1984, and has since reviewed the subject regularly with particular regard to the exposure of people at work. Despite the steady increase in number of cases of HIV infection in the community, the risk of occupational transmission remains extremely low.

A new ACDP publication on protection against blood-borne infections (HIV and hepatitis) in the workplace is planned for publication in 1995, and will supersede earlier guidance issued in 1990[26]. The new edition will widen the scope of the guidance to include some other prominent infection hazards that may be transmitted in the same way, particularly hepatitis B and certain other blood-borne viruses.

Health care

In health care settings, additional occupational health issues are raised by the need to prevent staff who might be carriers of certain infections from posing a risk to vulnerable patients. Close liaison between the occupational health service and infection control teams should ensure that there are appropriate policies for immunisation of staff, prevention and management of sharps injuries, and the identification of staff who may be infected or colonised with organisms such as methicillin-resistant *Staphylococcus aureus* or *Salmonella*. In 1993, the UK Health Departments published guidelines on protecting health care workers and patients from hepatitis B[27], and in 1994 updated guidance on the management of HIV-infected health care workers[28].

Occupational zoonoses

Zoonoses are infections that are transmitted from animals to humans. The incidence of occupational zoonoses in the UK is not known. Available data indicate that many are rare - particularly classic occupational zoonoses such as brucellosis and anthrax; for example, only seven cases of occupationally acquired anthrax have been reported in the last 10 years. Zoonoses such as cryptosporidiosis, however, are far from uncommon. This parasitic organism is transmitted by the faecal-oral route and is found in a range of animals, particularly young cattle and sheep, but it is not known how many cases are acquired by direct contact with animals and what proportion of these are occupationally acquired[29].

It is also important to recognise the range of occupations involved and the risk of indirect spread, such as spread of debris from bedding, as well as direct handling of animals. For example, avian chlamydiosis can affect taxidermists and building tradesmen as well as bird-keepers and pet-shop workers. Most cases of leptospirosis in the UK are not associated with rats or rat urine (*Leptospira icterohaemorrhagiae*) but with cattle (*L. hardjo*) - though the latter generally causes a milder illness.

For some zoonoses, the low incidence reflects steps taken to prevent workers acquiring infection - such as simple hygiene advice and the provision of adequate washing facilities, provision of protective clothing and immunisation. In others, such as brucellosis, the low incidence reflects eradication programmes in animals. Some groups of workers are issued with medical contact cards to assist doctors in making a rapid diagnosis.

Although there is no epidemiological evidence to suggest that occupational exposure to any of the transmissible spongiform encephalopathy agents (human or animal) has resulted in any cases of Creutzfeldt-Jakob disease (CJD) in the UK or worldwide, the ACDP issued guidance as a precautionary measure to protect workers from what remains at present a theoretical risk[30].

Genetically modified organisms

Regulations are in place in the UK to control the contained use and deliberate release of genetically modified organisms for commercial and research purposes, and are concerned with protecting human health and safety and the environment.

Although DH has no statutory responsibility, it has input at both national and European level to ensure that public health and health care interests are considered and protected. The Department has assessors on the Advisory Committee on Genetic Modification and the Advisory Committee on Releases to the Environment, and advises HSE and the Department of the Environment specifically on applications with health care implications.

(iv) Work-related psychosocial risks and ill-health

Studies of minor psychiatric morbidity in working populations indicate a high prevalence of between 270-370 per 1,000 employees[31]. During periods of occupational instability, such as labour disputes or threatened redundancies, rates may be significantly higher[32]. Minor psychiatric disorder is a major determinant of sickness absence, and is the second most common cause of absences lasting more than 21 days[33]. It is also at least as important as occupational attitudes in determining labour turnover[34]. Within the workplace, people suffering from mental health problems work less effectively and their relationships with colleagues and customers may be impaired[31]. The stigma that still attaches to mental health problems makes it difficult accurately to assess the total cost to industry, although one estimate places the annual cost at £26 billion[35].

Although personal or inherited characteristics may influence the risk of developing mental health problems, most mental health problems encountered in the workplace arise as a result of excessive or prolonged pressure or demands on individuals. Such pressures can arise from all domains of life, such as family life or personal relationships. Some, however, arise as a result of work. Certain characteristics of jobs and the working environment have proved to be stressful and potentially harmful to mental health[36]:

- organisational function and culture (with lack of management support and poor communication);

- conflict or ambiguity in role in organisation;

- job insecurity or uncertainty;

- lack of discretion or control over work;

- interpersonal relationships at work;

- home/work interface;

- design of task (eg, repetitive or fragmented work);

- underload or overload;

- unpredictable, long, or shift work schedules; and

- aggression and violence.

However, factors within the workplace and other areas of daily living can also act as sources of support and protect individuals from potentially adverse effects of demands elsewhere.

Although a great deal is known about methods to reduce mental ill-health at work, a survey by the Confederation of British Industry (CBI) and DH in 1991 showed that although 94% of respondent employers thought that mental illness should be of concern to their organisation, only 12% had a company policy on mental health[37]. DH issued its own policy on mental health in 1994.

Work-related risks to mental health are part of employers' broad responsibilities under health and safety law. The HSE has undertaken extensive research into occupational stress and prepared broad guidance for employers, designed to raise awareness of the issue and to clarify employers' responsibilities in this area, to be published in Spring 1995.

As part of the Health of the Nation strategy, DH has also been working to increase employers' awareness of the issues and to encourage them to take appropriate action. To ensure co-ordination of such strategies, DH convened the Mental Health at Work Inter-Agency Group in January. This replaced an informal working group which had existed for some years, and is composed of other Government Departments, the HSE, relevant advisory bodies (such as the Health Education Authority), and organisations representing employers (such as the CBI) and employees (such as the Trades Union Congress).

DH co-sponsored conferences in mental health at work in 1991[37] and 1993[31], and has held information stands at large conferences for employers in 1992, 1993 and 1994. Because of increasing concern about levels of mental ill-health among agricultural workers, DH held a stand on rural stress at the Royal Agricultural Show in July 1994.

To reach a wider audience, DH produced an information leaflet *A guide to mental health in the workplace*[38] for firms with more than 500 employees as part of the public information strategy on mental health in 1993. *ABC of mental health in the workplace*[39] - a resource pack for firms with 50-500 employees which provided key facts on mental health, methods of preventing and tackling mental health problems, and references to further information produced by the member organisations of the Mental Health at Work Inter-Agency Group - was issued in 1994.

(v) Rural issues

The countryside is not always considered a workplace, but agricultural and other rural workers may be exposed to a wide range of occupational health and safety risks, and this is reflected in mortality statistics[12]. Accidents due to falls from height and injury by cattle are of particular concern. There is a need for greater awareness of health matters. One issue which has recently attracted a lot of attention is the use of organophosphates as insecticides in sheep dipping solutions, particularly concern over the possibility of long-term effects (see page 200).

Other health risks include intoxication by oxides of nitrogen from silage; handling other pesticides and chemicals; hypersensitivity lung disorders from exposure to moulds and fungi; noise-induced deafness from operating heavy machinery; zoonoses from animal husbandry; musculo-skeletal disorders from heavy lifting and tractor vibration; and dermatitis from plants, chemicals, photosensitivity or physical trauma. One of the great difficulties is obtaining accurate incidence data on these conditions, because of under-reporting and other factors associated with the nature of the agricultural industry. This limits the likely effectiveness of targeted preventive effort, particularly where it is most needed. Much of the morbidity and mortality associated with agriculture can be prevented. In 1993, DH organised a meeting, in conjunction with the Royal Agricultural Society and the Royal Institute of Public Health and Hygiene, at which some of these occupational health issues were discussed.

References

1. Health and Safety Executive. *Surveillance of people exposed to health risks at work*. London: HMSO, 1990.
2. Office of Population Censuses and Surveys, Health and Safety Executive. *Occupational health: decennial supplement (Series: DS no. 10)*. London: HMSO (in press).
3. International Agency for Research on Cancer. *IARC Monographs on the evaluation of carcinogenic risks to humans: an updating of Monographs vols 1-42*. Lyon: International Agency for Research on Cancer, 1987 (Suppl 7).
4. Doll R, Peto J. *The causes of cancer*. Oxford: Oxford University Press, 1982.
5. Office of Population Censuses and Surveys. *Labour Force Survey 1990*. London: HMSO, 1993.
6. Sallie BS, Ross DJ, Meredith SK, McDonald JC. SWORD '93 surveillance of work-related and occupational respiratory disease in the UK. *Occup Med* 1994; **44:** 177-82.
7. Health and Safety Executive. *Preventing asthma at work: how to control respiratory sensitisers*. London: Health and Safety Executive, 1994.
8. Venables KM, Topping MD, Nunn AJ, Howe W, Newman Taylor AJ. Immunologic and functional consequences of chemical (tetrachlorophthalic anhydride) induced asthma after 4 years of avoidance of exposure. *J Allergy Clin Immunol* 1987; **80:** 212-8.
9. Cullinan P, Lowson D, Nieuwenhuijsen MJ, et al. Work related symptoms, sensitisation and estimated exposure to workers not previously exposed to flour. *Occup Environ Med* 1994; **51:** 579-83.
10. Cullinan P, Lowson D, Nieuwenhuijsen MJ et al. Work-related symptoms, sensitisation and estimated exposure in workers not previously exposed to laboratory rats. *Occup Rev Med* 1994; **51:** 589-92.
11. Health and Safety Commission. *Health and safety statistics: supplement to 1993/94 annual report*. London: Health and Safety Executive, 1994; 54-6.
12. Health and Safety Commission. *Health and safety statistics: statistical supplement to the 1993/94 annual report*. London: HMSO, 1994; 60.
13. Benn T. Estimation of the prevalence of hand-arm vibration syndrome in Great Britain. *Proc Inst Acoustics* 1993; **15:** 463-70.
14. *Noise at Work Regulations 1989*. London: HMSO, 1989.
15. Mills KB, Bion R, Saunders DC. In: Raffle PAB, Adams PH, Baxter PJ, Lee WR, eds. *Hunter's diseases of occupations, 8th edn*. London: Edward Arnold, 1994.
16. Sagan LA, Kheifets LI. In: Raffle PAB, Adams PH, Baxter PJ, Lee WR, eds. *Hunter's diseases of occupations, 8th edn*. London: Edward Arnold, 1994.
17. National Radiological Protection Board. *Health effects related to the use of visual display units: report of an Advisory Group on non-ionising radiation*. Oxford: National Radiological Protection Board, 1994.
18. National Radiological Protection Board. *Electromagnetic fields and the risk of cancer: report of the Advisory Group on Non-ionising Radiation*. Oxford: National Radiological Protection Board, 1994.
19. National Radiological Protection Board. *Electromagnetic fields and the risk of cancer: supplementary report by the Advisory Group on Non-ionising Radiation*. Oxford: National Radiological Protection Board, 1994.
20. Advisory Committee on Dangerous Pathogens. *Categorisation of pathogens 1984 according to the hazards and categories of containment*. London: Health and Safety Commission, 1984.
21. Advisory Committee on Dangerous Pathogens. *Categorisation of pathogens 1990 according to the hazards and categories of containment*. London: Health and Safety Commission, 1990.
22. *Health and Safety at Work etc. Act 1974*. London: HMSO, 1974
23. *Control of Substances Hazardous to Health (COSHH) Regulations 1988*. London: HMSO, 1988.
24. *Control of Substances Hazardous to Health (COSHH) Regulations 1994*. London: HMSO, 1994.
25. Department of Health. *Guidance for clinical health care workers: protection against infection with HIV and hepatitis viruses*. London: Department of Health, 1990.
26. Advisory Committee on Dangerous Pathogens. *HIV - the causative agent of AIDS and related conditions: second revision of guidelines*. London: Health and Safety Commission, 1990.

27. Department of Health. *Protecting health care workers and patients from hepatitis B*. Heywood (Lancashire): Department of Health, 1993 (Health Service Guidelines: HSG(93)40).
28. Department of Health. *AIDS/HIV infected health care workers: guidance on the management of infected health care workers*. Heywood (Lancashire): Department of Health, 1994 (Health Service Guidelines: HSG (94)16).
29. Health and Safety Executive. *The occupational zoonoses*. London: Health and Safety Executive, 1993.
30. Advisory Committee on Dangerous Pathogens. *Precautions for work with human and animal transmissible spongiform encephalopathies*. London: HMSO, 1994.
31. Jenkins R. *Defining the problem: stress, depression and anxiety: causes, prevalence and consequences*. In: Jenkins R, Warman D, eds. *Promoting mental health policies in the workplace*. London: HMSO, 1993.
32. Macbride A, Lancee W, Freeman SJJ. The psychosocial impact of a labour dispute. *J Occup Psychol* 1981; **54:** 125-33.
33. Stansfeld S, Feeney A, Head J, Canner R, North F, Marmot M. Sickness absence for psychiatric illness: the Whitehall II Study. *Soc Sci Med* (in press)
34. Jenkins R. Minor psychiatric morbidity and labour turnover. *Br J Indust Med* 1985; **42:** 534-9.
35. National Association for Staff Support. *The costs of stress and the costs and benefits of stress management*. London: Royal College of Nursing, 1992.
36. Cox T. *Stress research and stress management: putting theory to work*. London: Health and Safety Executive, 1993 (HSE Contract Research Report 61/1993).
37. Banham J. The costs of mental ill health to business. In: Jenkins R, Coney N, eds. *Prevention of mental ill health at work*. London: HMSO, 1992.
38. Department of Health. *A guide to mental health in the workplace*. London: Department of Health, 1993.
39. Department of Health. *ABC of mental health in the workplace*. London: Department of Health, 1994.

(g)   Effects of health on work

A relatively small number of jobs have specific criteria for medical standards of fitness to help to ensure that employees carry out tasks safely, without undue harm to themselves or others. For such jobs the safety of the general public is often the primary interest, rather than that of the employee, such as for airline pilots or drivers of heavy goods vehicles[1,2]. In most types of work there are no clearly defined criteria for fitness on medical grounds[3].

Judgment of an individual's suitability for work may differ widely and employer, employee and medical adviser may hold various opinions on the matter. Opinion may also differ among the different medical practitioners involved in a particular case. While a number of issues need to be considered in the assessment, it is often the nature and significance of the workplace risks - and their acceptability - which are critical to the decision. These can be reconciled in many cases following careful evaluation of the circumstances: a proper assessment of the working environment and duties involved, and a health assessment which is appropriate to the type of work to be done. In many cases, changes to the working environment or ways in which the job is done can overcome problems for individual workers who have particular needs.

While the risks of the job need to be considered, in practice one of the main purposes of an informed assessment of fitness is to reduce unnecessary restrictions being imposed on employability. Many people with chronic ill-health and disabilities can work safely and productively in environments where lay opinion may suggest otherwise.

Two particular challenges can be mentioned: the employment prospects of people with mental illness, and of those with learning disorders. Most people with mental health problems recover completely, through a planned return to work in consultation with an individual's carers, occupational health specialists or disability employment advisers is generally advisable. Evaluation of potential stress factors within the workplace, specific action to reduce them and the provision of general support in the early stages will promote a smoother return to productive work. Patients with learning disabilities often integrate successfully into open employment with minimal difficulty. Many become able and conscientious workers given time, even though acquisition of new skills may be relatively slow in the early days. For some, accompanying medical conditions or drug therapy may pose additional problems and careful assessment of occupational implications is required.

Employers, general practitioners and others can obtain expert advice from placement, assessment and counselling teams, through local job centres, and from publications of patient groups and voluntary organisations[4,5]. The 'Access to Work' scheme, launched in 1994, provides practical advice and financial assistance for employers to help them to employ people with disabilities, by making alterations to work premises or providing support staff to assist those with hearing or visual impairments.

References

1. *Motor Vehicles (Driver Licences) Regulations 1987.* London: HMSO, 1987.
2. *Motor Vehicles (Driver Licences) Regulations 1987 as amended 1990.* London: HMSO, 1990.
3. Cox RAF, Edwards FC, McCallum RI, eds. *Fitness for work: the medical aspects.* Oxford: Oxford University Press (in press).
4. Health and Safety Executive. *Health aspects of job placement and rehabilitation: advice to employers.* London: HMSO, 1989 (HSE Guidance note: HS23).
5. Kettle M, Massie B. *Employer's guide to disabilities, 2nd edn.* Cambridge: Woodhead-Faulkener, 1986.

(h)   Health promotion

The WHO has defined health promotion as "the process of enabling people to increase control over and thereby improve their health"[1]. The workforce is a useful population for health promotion activity.

A Task Force for health promotion in the workplace was established as part of the Health of the Nation strategy[2] in November 1992, consisting of representatives from the CBI, the HEA, DH, the HSE, the Trades Union Congress, the Faculty of Occupational Medicine and others. A steering group has been set up to monitor progress on implementation of the recommendations made by the Task Force. The Health of the Nation strategy has reinforced the need to strengthen local alliances between the NHS, environmental health departments, professional bodies and charitable organisations.

Employers can contribute by developing and implementing workplace health promotion policies, guided by competent professionals, and they may benefit from increased employee morale, less absenteeism and staff turnover, and increased performance and productivity.

References

1. World Health Organization. Ottowa Charter for Health Promotion. *Health Promotion* 1986; **i:** i-v.
2. Department of Health. *The Health of the Nation: a strategy for health in England.* London: HMSO, 1992 (Cm. 1986).

(i)   Occupational health services

Occupational health services (OHSs) offer a specialist advisory service to promote health and safety for management and employees alike. Their use is not compulsory, but employers are required to seek competent advice to identify and to meet their occupational health needs. Larger firms may prefer to set up a comprehensive in-house occupational health service; smaller firms can join a service that provides shared facilities to a number of employers. OHS staffing varies according to need but can include occupational health doctors and nurses, occupational hygienists and other specialists. A recent survey[1] showed that employment of doctors and/or nurses by private sector firms (employing more than eleven people) had increased from 5.5% to 14% over a period of 15 years, but the percentage of the labour force covered had fallen from 52% to 34%, because of a change in employment structure (mainly the growth in the small business sector). Occupational health departments in the NHS could broaden their role, once policies and management systems have been fully established for their own direct responsibilities, and provide help for small and medium-sized businesses, or referral clinics for use by medical practitioners who identify or suspect work-related illness in their patients.

Over the past 20 years, the role of occupational health services has been re-examined. Greater emphasis is now placed on advisory rather than treatment services; giving advice on prevention as well as protection; health surveillance; and multi-disciplinary expertise. Employers now seek increasingly flexible services to meet the needs revealed by risk assessment.

A conference on the value of occupational health services in December, organised by the Faculty of Occupational Medicine of the Royal College of Physicians and the Institute of Health Services Management was addressed by the Secretary of State for Health.

Reference

1.   Bunt K. *Occupational health provision at work.* London: HMSO, 1993 (HSE contract research report no. 57/1993).

(j)   Ethics and confidentiality

It is vital that the impartiality, integrity and confidentiality of occupational health services is maintained and recognised by other health care personnel as well as by employees and managers. Information that is accessible to management and enforcing authorities should be handled separately from confidential clinical records on individuals. Guidance on ethical matters for occupational physicians has been issued by the Faculty of Occupational Medicine[1].

Reference

1.   Faculty of Occupational Medicine, Royal College of Physicians of London. *Guidance on ethics for occupational physicians, 4th edn.* London: Royal College of Physicians, 1993.

(k)   Health of NHS staff

The physical and mental health and well-being of employees should be a major concern to all managers. Risks will vary in different parts of the service but policies should address the health risks from infectious agents such as hepatitis B and HIV; chemical hazards such as disinfectants and latex allergy; physical hazards such as radiation and lasers and manual handling; violence to staff; stress; and other problems. These issues are not confined to clinical staff and a suitable assessment will highlight the groups at risk.

Health and safety risk management is an essential task for all parts of the NHS to protect the health of staff, patients and others who could be affected. Accurate identification and prioritisation of workplace risks is needed for good management and effective control. In 1993, DH produced a risk management manual for health care organisations which outlined a structured approach to the complex problems likely to be encountered[1]. More specific guidance on successful health and safety management has been prepared by the HSC's Health Services Advisory Committee and will be helpful to health service directors and managers[2].

A healthy workforce is essential for the NHS to provide high-quality health care and to improve the health of the population. The 'Health at Work in the NHS' (HAWNHS) initiative, launched in 1992, was set up by the NHS Executive to support the national strategy for health in England[3]. It seeks to pursue all of the Health of the Nation targets in each NHS workplace, to enlist healthier NHS staff as ambassadors for the promotion of healthier lifestyles, and to provide an example to other employers. The Health Education Authority (HEA) was commissioned to help to develop and to promote a programme of action. During its second year, the project researched sickness absence, mental health, communicable diseases, training and communication; issued guidance on existing good practice; sponsored regional events to share information and best practice; and set up a database of HAWNHS contacts. NHS employers were alerted to the scope of HAWNHS and the potential for occupational health services to help to improve cost-effectiveness through the reduction of sickness absence and accidents, as well as improving the quality of patient care and other services through enhanced staff morale[4].

The Department has helped to set up clinical audit projects which may be used as models throughout the NHS; DH funding has been administered by the Association of NHS Occupational Physicians for projects looking at aspects of pre-employment health assessment and long-term sickness absence. It is hoped that these will help to stimulate similar initiatives on other topics.

In 1994, the HEA commissioned the then Institute of Manpower Studies to establish baseline data on sickness absence, staff wastage and accidents in the NHS. The survey showed significant differences in reported sickness absence rates in different parts of the service, reflecting differences in activities of the occupational groups employed, staff attendance practices operated by management and other factors. It also highlighted the need for better information to be collected on the causes and location of accidents and cases of ill-health.

References

1. NHS Management Executive. *Risk management in the NHS.* Heywood (Lancashire): Department of Health, 1993.
2. Health and Safety Commission, Health Services Advisory Committee. *Management of health and safety in the health services: information for directors and managers.* London: HMSO, 1994.
3. Department of Health. *The Health of the Nation: a strategy for health in England.* London: HMSO, 1992 (Cm. 1986).
4. NHS Executive. *Occupational health services for NHS staff.* Heywood (Lancashire): Department of Health, 1994 (Health Service Guidelines: HSG(94)51).

(l)   Responsibilities and training

Occupational health services have independent professional status and should report to senior management. Those responsible for running an occupational health service should have appropriate specialist qualifications, depending on the type of service provided. Effective implementation of risk assessment, risk management, and surveillance requires specialist skills. Several options for training of health and safety professionals are now available. Trained and competent professionals will contribute to improvements in the standard of health in the workplace.

For occupational physicians, a series of approved training posts leading to membership of the Faculty of Occupational Medicine is the route for specialist training. The required period of general professional training has been reduced to two years, although the need for four years in an approved occupational medicine post remains unchanged. In 1994, the Faculty of Occupational Medicine introduced a new Diploma in Occupational Medicine to cater for other physicians who require non-specialist training in the discipline. Nurses may train to receive a Certificate or Diploma in occupational health nursing. Discussions between occupational health and safety groups have also taken place on standards of competence, with a view to the introduction of national vocational qualifications (NVQs) for occupational health and safety practitioners. It is anticipated that health and safety activities organised under continuing development programmes will involve universities, industry, the health service and professional organisations nationally and internationally. Other groups with important responsibilities in health and safety at work - safety officers, occupational hygienists, ergonomists and others - undertake specialised training and are part of the multi-disciplinary occupational health and safety team.

(m)   Audit in occupational health

As in other areas of professional practice, the cost-benefit and effectiveness of procedures and interventions in occupational health must be evaluated. Audit of the structure, process or outcome of practice assists the development of improved clinical standards and guidelines, contributes to continuing professional development and helps to meet the needs of the client or user of the service. Audit may yield benefits in terms of education and practice, although it does not necessarily help to bridge gaps in existing knowledge or skills[1]. Many of the issues are likely to benefit from a multi-disciplinary approach in which development of an integrated team is vital[2].

Pre-employment screening in the health service has been audited in a DH-funded project which found a wide variation in the procedures used[3]. Further analysis of the reasons for questions being included in pre-employment questionnaires should help occupational health services to review their approach to pre-employment screening and to introduce appropriate changes.

The effectiveness of occupational health services in contributing to the management of absence attributed to sickness is under evaluation in the NHS and in several industries. Audit of the delivery of occupational health services and the contribution which they can make to helping an organisation reach its objectives is now established practice in some organisations and occupational health departments. This process should encourage the exchange of information and examples of good practice in industry and the NHS on the delivery of efficient and effective occupational health care. A report with guidance on audit and quality in occupational medicine will be available from the Faculty of Occupational Medicine of the Royal College of Physicians of London in Spring 1995.

References

1. Agius RM, Lee RJ, Symington IS, Riddle HFV, Seaton A. Audit of occupational health consultation records. *Occup Med* 1994; **44:** 151-7.
2. Department of Health. *Working for patients: medical audit.* London: HMSO, 1989.
3. Whitaker S, Aw TC. Audit of pre-employment assessments by occupational health departments in the National Health Service. *Occup Med* (in press).

(n)   Research

The HSE's occupational health research programme is informed by the priority areas and objectives identified by the HSC's health risk reviews. Much research effort is aimed at developing more effective control measures; understanding people's perception of health risks; and obtaining better information on the scale, pattern and nature of illness and on the key causative agents. Research into subjects such as occupational asthma, psychological hazards and musculo-skeletal disorders is a high priority, and more sensitive means are being sought to detect the effects of exposure to toxic materials. New research will complement studies already under way or recently completed in these areas, which include: research into exposure/response relations for respiratory sensitisers; work on the effectiveness of organisational interventions for occupational stress; and an investigation of the occupational factors associated with upper limb soft tissue disorders in keyboard operators.

Both the HSE and the recently established British Occupational Health Research Foundation (BOHRF) are not only encouraging the development of a list of priorities but also setting out the long-term challenges that should be addressed. For example, the HSE are funding a series of workshops to identify research questions in key areas. For its part, the BOHRF will set up a complementary series of workshops and seek industrial partners with specific interest in a given topic to help to fund such projects. Research proposals will then be invited by competitive tender with funds increasingly diverted to projects which concentrate on key questions, to ensure that money spent on research is clearly focused on practical problems of recognised concern in industry and commerce.

A survey of senior occupational health staff in a wide range of organisations employed the Delphi technique to identify priority issues and achieved a general consensus on important areas for research[1].

The research panel of the Association of NHS Occupational Physicians reviews research proposals relevant to occupational health in the NHS. Current areas of research interest include exposure to glutaraldehyde, dermatitis from latex gloves and stress in hospital staff. Occupational health departments within the NHS and local authorities have also developed ideas and opportunities for practice-based research. One area currently being explored is to research the extent of occupational ill-health seen in general practice and to develop referral mechanisms for preventive action.

Increased attention has been paid in North America and Europe alike to the establishment of research priorities. Whilst this process is as yet incomplete, the general consensus seems to be that musculo-skeletal problems (such as back pain and work-related upper limb disorders), asthma, injuries and accidents, and dermatitis figure prominently in most surveys. The development of audit procedures, the environmental impact of industry and stress-related disorders are other broad areas of concern.

Reference

1. Harrington JM. Research priorities in occupational medicine: a survey of United Kingdom medical opinion by the Delphi technique. *Occup Environ Med* 1994; **51:** 289-94.

(o)   Future developments and emerging issues

(i)   Strategic health risk reviews

The HSC and HSE recently set up a major review of ten principal occupational health risks. This review identified strategic priorities and set out proposals for action on each health risk, which are now being put into effect - for example through published guidance, publicity initiatives and inspection campaigns.

Some common themes which emerged from the health risk review were the need to:

-    develop further knowledge of the epidemiology of occupational ill-health;

-    tackle certain risks by working with suppliers and manufacturers (eg, by encouraging the substitution of safer alternatives for certain hazardous products);

-    make sustained efforts to improve industry's management of health problems;

- produce guidance on common health problems with an emphasis on practical methods to deal with them; *and*

- redirect research into ill-health to concentrate on behavioural studies (eg, what affects perception of risk) and the development of practical techniques for prevention.

(ii)   *Reproductive health*

Hazards to reproductive health are commanding increased attention. HSE has established a £0.5 million research programme to investigate whether exposure to chemicals is affecting male fertility and whether suitable biomarkers can be identified for sub-clinical health effects. HSE is also contributing to an EC collaborative study to investigate industries where there is the potential for exposure to reproductive toxins. A National Teratology Information Service has recently been established at the Northern and Yorkshire Regional Drug and Therapeutics Centre in Newcastle, which will support NHS interests in this field and contribute to research and educational activities.

(iii)   *Genetic screening*

Certain inherited traits may increase the risk of acquiring occupational disease. For example, deficiency of the enzyme glucose-6-phosphate dehydrogenase in red blood cells increases the risk of haemolysis on exposure to trinitrotoluene[1]. Genetic screening tests could potentially be used as part of pre-employment health assessment to determine fitness for a particular type of work. While there are relatively few reliable tests for 'susceptibility' to specific conditions, advances in molecular biology and genetic screening may, however, lead to identifiable genetic dispositions for occupational risks. Such knowledge could lead to measures being taken to protect employees. However, such applications raise important legal and ethical issues which have not yet been resolved.

Genetic monitoring is a form of periodic surveillance of workers in which genetic material in body fluid is tested for evidence of adverse effects due to occupational exposures. This could be applied as a screening test in industries where carcinogens are handled - for example a technique being developed by workers in Oxford to detect very early malignant change in cells exfoliated in body fluids by CD44 gene activity[2].

(iv)   *Environmental issues*

Occupational health professionals' broad knowledge of clinical medicine, human factors, toxicology and epidemiology can be invaluable in furthering our understanding of environmental risks to the public health and in how to respond appropriately to them. In March, the Faculties of Occupational Medicine and Public Health Medicine of the Royal College of Physicians of London set up a joint Standing Group on the Environment to act as a focus of professional medical interest and advice and to stimulate future debate and research. The Department supports the initiative and is represented on the group. Occupational health is integrated into the broader environmental strategy of WHO's Environmental Health Action Plan for Europe. The UK is one of six pilot countries currently drafting national action plans, with the Department of the Environment taking the lead on preparation. A discussion document should be published during 1995. Other countries will be able to benefit from the UK's preparation before drafting their own plans in advance of the Third European Conference on Environment and Health in 1999.

(v)   *International issues*

Occupational health is not just a national issue, and the UK has a lot to learn from, and contribute to, international debate. A Joint European Committee, representing the Society and the Faculty of Occupational Medicine, the BMA and the Joint Committee on Higher Medical Training has organised meetings for representatives from all Member States of the EC. The recently established European Association for Schools of Occupational Medicine provides a forum to compare and co-ordinate education and training activities between the UK and other European countries. A European network of occupational health nursing educators and teachers (EUROHNET) hold meetings and workshops to exchange ideas and information for the mutual benefit of participating countries. A Scientific Committee of the International Congress on Occupational Health (ICOH) will hold an Occupational Health Services Research and Evaluation conference in Glasgow in November 1995, and other planned ventures include an ICOH Health Care Workers Conference in 1997.

(vi)   *The way ahead*

The protection of health of people at work is a subject which, in one way or another, affects us all. Much of the burden of work-related ill-health is preventable, and there is a need for greater appreciation of the risks and better understanding of how to manage them effectively. Health surveillance may be needed where there is evidence of residual risk. Periodic or special medical examination of employees may be required and workers should be adequately trained.

Responsibility for ensuring the health of its workers must be a core management responsibility of any organisation. Management systems should incorporate procedures to identify hazards, to assess risks and to implement and maintain all necessary control measures. Guidance and support will often need to be sought from technical experts and occupational health practitioners with the relevant training and experience to address the needs of the business and of individual employees.

The rapid development and implementation of technological advances in industry increases, rather than diminishes, the need to protect and value our human resources. Doctors and other health care professionals should consider what contribution they may be able to make to prevention of work-related illness. Identification or suspicion of an occupational disease or work-related component to a multi-factorial disorder in an individual patient should prompt further inquiries and consultation with an occupational health specialist, so that further investigation can be arranged to prevent others from being similarly affected. Increasing expectations for healthy, satisfying lives, the complexity and changing risks within the workplace today and increasing recognition of the value of occupational health provision all emphasise the importance of ensuring health for all in the workplace.

References

1. Djerassi LSS, Vitany I. Haemolytic episode in G6PD deficient workers exposed to TNT. *Br J Indust Med* 1975; **32:** 54-58.
2. Matsumura Y, Hanbury D, Smith J, Tarin D. Non-invasive detection of malignancy by identification of unusual CD44 gene activity in exfoliated cancer cells. *BMJ* 1994: **308:** 619-24.

CHAPTER 5

HEALTH CARE

(a)   Needs, effectiveness and outcomes

(i)   *Health needs assessment*

The assessment of health needs continues to develop as a core activity of District Health Authorities (DHAs). Considerable activity is taking placed locally, led by public health departments. The series of epidemiologically based needs reviews, described in earlier Reports[1,2], is being extended to cover: accident and emergency, gynaecology, child and adolescent mental health services, terminal and palliative care, rehabilitation, sexually transmitted diseases, dermatology, back pain, breast cancer, and the health of ethnic minority groups. During the year, a compilation of epidemiologically based needs assessment reviews was published[3], covering: diabetes mellitus; renal disease; stroke and cerebrovascular disease; lower respiratory disease; coronary heart disease (CHD); colorectal cancer; cancer of the lung; total hip replacement; total knee replacement; cataract surgery; hernia repair; varicose vein treatments; prostatectomy for benign prostatic hyperplasia; mental illness; dementia; alcohol misuse; drug abuse; people with learning difficulties; community child health services (community-based services, services for disabled children, and child mental health: mild psychological pathology); and family planning, abortion and fertility services.

The Department of Health (DH) is also reviewing this series to improve the usefulness of needs reviews in decision-making by DHAs, National Health Service (NHS) Trusts, and general practitioners (GPs), in the light of increasing emphasis on the role of the primary care team as a purchaser of care on the patient's behalf as well as being a provider of services.

(ii)   *Basic sources of information*

The Health Survey programme

The 1992 Health Survey for England report, the second in a series of annual surveys designed to monitor trends in the nation's health, appeared early in 1994[4]; the report of the 1993 Survey will be published early in 1995. The 1993 and 1994 Surveys ran throughout the calendar years and each included approximately 17,000 individuals; like previous Surveys, they are focused on cardiovascular disease and associated risk factors, but will also enable regional variations to be assessed. The larger sample size will provide more precise estimates for sub-groups of the population and generally increase the precision of all estimates. The 1995 Health Survey will also include data from children and deal with other important health issues - such as asthma, accidents and disability.

In 1993, DH commissioned the Office of Population Censuses and Surveys (OPCS) to carry out a series of national psychiatric morbidity surveys which were completed in 1994. They comprised a survey of 10,000 households; a survey of institutions; a supplementary sample of people with psychosis; and a survey of the roofless and homeless. The results from these surveys will be published in a series of bulletins and reports. The first bulletin, produced in December 1994[5], reported the main findings on prevalence: 16% of adults had suffered a neurotic disorder in the previous week and 0.4% had suffered from a psychotic disorder in the past year. The results from these surveys will help to underpin policy and provide information for progress in the Health of the Nation mental illness key area. The data will be subsequently placed in the Economic and Social Research Council data archive during 1995. The methodology is available from DH for purchasers and others who wish to use it for more detailed local surveys to inform local needs assessments.

Further work on various topics has also been commissioned by DH, including surveys of diet and nutrition (see page 69).

Public Health Information Strategy

In 1990, DH set up the Public Health Information Strategy (PHIS) programme to ensure that it collects the information required to support the Department's public health objectives in the most cost-effective way. The final report of the strategy was delivered in 1992. Since then, the strategy team has addressed a wide range of individual topics including mental health, the health of ethnic minority groups, maternity and child health, and the production of overviews of public health information. Work on accidents has been endorsed by the Inter-Departmental Accidents Prevention Task Force and will be taken forward during 1995.

(iii)   National confidential enquiries

The Reports for 1992[6] and 1993[7] described the purposes of confidential enquiry, summarised the principles of the methods used, and outlined the progress of the five national confidential enquiries.

Progress was maintained during 1994. The report of the Confidential Enquiries into Maternal Deaths in the United Kingdom (UK) (see page 146) was published in January[8], and an interim report of the Confidential Inquiry into Homicides and Suicides by Mentally Ill People (see page 142) was published in August[9]. The enquiries into Peri-operative Deaths, Stillbirths and Deaths in Infancy, and Counselling for Genetic Disorders continued to collect and to analyse data for reports due to be published in 1995.

DH also made preparations for a workshop, to be held early in 1995, to consider how better use might be made of confidential enquiries to improve the effectiveness of the NHS. In particular, the workshop will consider how the conduct of such enquiries can be improved, and how a systematic approach to the implementation of recommendations from confidential enquiries could be developed.

(iv) *Quality of service and effectiveness of care*

The transfer of good research evidence into changed and improved health services is a key goal for the Department, reflected in priorities and planning guidance for the NHS in 1995/96[10]. A number of initiatives contribute to this process. Guidance issued in December 1993 to purchasers and providers listed sources of information on clinical effectiveness[11]; the NHS Executive sought feedback from purchasers and providers through a series of national workshops, and took into account other work on improving clinical effectiveness - such as the work undertaken by the then Oxford Regional Health Authority (RHA) 'Getting Research into Practice and Purchasing' (GRiPP) project. Further information about sources of information on clinical effectiveness, including high quality clinical guidelines, was issued in September[12] .

Overall clinical effectiveness can only be improved in the long term, and DH is working widely with professionals and managers on such a strategy to achieve improved clinical effectiveness. The Clinical Outcomes Group (COG), jointly chaired by the Chief Medical and Chief Nursing Officers, is the national professional steering mechanism for this work, and has established various sub-groups. The COG also oversees the strategic development of clinical audit, which seeks to improve the quality and outcome of patient care through clinicians and other health care professionals examining their procedures and comparing them with best practice.

In February, DH published a series of detailed reports on the programmes for medical audit in the hospital and community health services[13], clinical audit in the nursing and physiotherapy professions[14], medical audit in primary care[15] and the audit activities of the medical Royal Colleges[16]. These reports covered the first three years of the audit programmes from 1989/90 to 1992/93, and were compiled from reports received from the fourteen RHAs over that period.

The Clinical Accountability Service Planning and Evaluation group (CASPE) was also commissioned by DH to evaluate the development, progress and impact of audit in hospital care health services in England. The CASPE group published two reports during 1994 - *The development of audit: findings of a national survey of healthcare provider units in England*[17] and *The role of the commissioner in audit*[18]. The survey's findings to date indicate that clinical audit has been firmly embedded in clinical practice and healthcare provision in the NHS, and that a good foundation for the future development of audit and quality improvement has been created.

(v) *National Casemix Office and NHS Centre for Coding and Classification*

National Casemix Office

The National Casemix Office has been set up to develop, maintain, issue and market patient grouping tools and classification methodologies for use in the NHS. Such groupings allow patient-based data to be aggregated in various ways to assist in analysis. One type of grouping is healthcare resource groups (HRGs) for use in costing, the contracting process and for internal resource management; the second version of this system was released in August. Other types of groupings, for example, health benefit groups (HBGs) enable analysis of epidemiological data to assist purchasers to define needs. The Office has close working relations with the NHS Centre for Coding and Classification, with whom it shares a supervisory board responsible for strategic guidance.

The current programme includes:

- development of HRGs in radiotherapy, psychiatry, geriatrics and accident and emergency medicine for release during 1995;

- development of HRGs and HBGs to help to negotiate and monitor community service contracts by Autumn 1995;

- casemix standardisation of health service indicators;

- development of HBGs to inform purchasing;

- provision of training in the use of casemix grouping methods;

- provision of a casemix database; *and*

- management of the co-ordination of community information projects.

NHS Centre for Coding and Classification

The NHS Centre for Coding and Classification (NHSCCC) continues to maintain and develop the Read codes - a computerised thesaurus of healthcare terms and one of the key projects of the information management and technology strategy for the NHS in England[19]. The NHSCCC also has new responsibility for healthcare classifications following the transfer of staff and functions from the Clinical Coding Support Unit. In November, the British Computer Society awarded one of its three gold medals to the NHSCCC for their technical achievement in creating version 3 of the Read Codes.

The main activities during the year include work to:

- ensure medical, nursing and allied professional support for Read Codes;

- implement the use of Read Codes in the NHS;

- develop further terms related to nursing, midwifery and health visiting and for other professions allied to medicine;

- support the implementation of the International Classification of Diseases version 10 (ICD-10) for national returns, with conversion tables between ICD-10 and its predecessor ICD-9; *and*

- development of a Read Codes 'stimulator' to illustrate how information technology can be applied to healthcare.

(vi) Clinical outcomes

Development of health outcome indicators

The first set of Population Health Outcome Indicators [20, 21], though well received, were based on currently available data, rather than being indicators that the NHS needed but which would entail new data collection. The Central Health Outcomes Unit (CHOU) has now commissioned work to develop a set of 'ideal' indicators, covering ten health topics over two years. An updated set of the first-phase indicators will be published as part of the Public Health Common Data Set in 1995 and the use of these indicators by health authorities, perhaps augmented from existing local data sources, will be evaluated over the following 12 months.

The development of new outcome indicators has been undertaken by Anglia and Oxford RHA. A workshop will be held in January 1995 to set out criteria for selection and to propose a shortlist of health topics for special attention. Asthma has already been used as a topic to pilot methods and approaches.

An NHS Executive Working Group recommended the construction of a composite population health outcome indicator to assist assessment of quality and effectiveness to set alongside the efficiency index. Its report suggested that a composite indicator could be derived from the population health outcomes indicator set by calculating and totalling the extent to which a health authority deviates from a standard or target value for each indicator. For this exercise, indicators would be presented in two ways:

- a cross-sector comparison by Health Authority; *and*

- a time series, showing relative improvements from the base year.

Work is in progress to produce sample composite indicators.

Clinical quality indicators

After inviting suggestions from the medical profession for indicators of clinical quality which could be included with NHS performance tables, a joint DH/Joint Consultants Committee Working Group was set up to recommend such indicators. The Department has commissioned a feasibility study of suggested indicators and produced sample data. An interim report will include recommendations for further development.

References

1. Department of Health. *On the State of the Public Health: the report of the Chief Medical Officer of the Department of Health for the year 1992.* London: HMSO, 1993; 107-9.
2. Department of Health. *On the State of the Public Health: the report of the Chief Medical Officer of the Department of Health for the year 1993.* London: HMSO, 1994; 113.

3. Stevens A, Raftery J, eds. *Health care needs asessment: the epidemiologically based needs assessment reviews (vols I and II)*. Oxford: Radcliffe Press, 1994.
4. Office of Population Censuses and Surveys. *Health Survey for England 1992*. London: HMSO, 1994.
5. Meltzer H. *The prevalence of psychiatric morbidity among adults aged 16-64, living in private households, in Great Britain*. London: Office of Population Censuses and Surveys, 1994 (OPCS Surveys of Psychiatric Morbidity in Great Britain; bulletin 1).
6. Department of Health. *On the State of the Public Health: the annual report of the Chief Medical Officer of the Department of Health for the year 1992*. London: HMSO, 1993; 109-10.
7. Department of Health. *On the State of the Public Health: the annual report of the Chief Medical Officer of the Department of Health for the year 1993*. London: HMSO, 1994; 115.
8. Department of Health, Welsh Office, Scottish Office Home and Health Department, Northern Ireland Department of Health and Social Services. *Report on Confidential Enquiries into Maternal Deaths in the United Kingdom 1988-90*. London: HMSO, 1994.
9. Steering Committee of the Confidential Inquiry into Homicides and Suicides by Mentally Ill People. *A preliminary report on homicide*. London: Steering Committee of the Confidential Inquiry into Homicides and Suicides, 1994.
10. Department of Health. *Priorities and planning guidance for the NHS 1995/96*. Heywood (Lancashire): Department of Health, 1994 (Executive Letter: EL(94)55).
11. Department of Health. *Improving clinical effectiveness*. Heywood (Lancashire): Department of Health, 1993 (Executive Letter: EL(93)115).
12. Department of Health. *Improving the effectiveness of the NHS*. Heywood (Lancashire): Department of Health, 1994 (Executive Letter: EL(94)74).
13. Department of Health. *Medical audit in the hospital and community health services*. Heywood (Lancashire): Department of Health, 1994.
14. Department of Health. *Clinical audit in the nursing and therapy professions*. Heywood (Lancashire): Department of Health, 1994.
15. Department of Health. *Medical audit in primary care*. Heywood (Lancashire): Department of Health, 1994.
16. Department of Health. *Medical audit in the Royal Colleges and their Faculties in the UK*. Heywood (Lancashire): Department of Health, 1994.
17. Buttery Y, Walshe K, Coles J, Bennett J. *The development of audit: findings of a national survey of healthcare provider units in England*. London: CASPE Research, 1994.
18. Rumsey M, Walshe K, Bennett J, Coles J. *The role of the commissioner in audit*. London: CASPE Research, 1994.
19. Department of Health. New national thesaurus. *CMO's Update* 1994; **4:** 1.
20. Department of Health. *Population health outcome indicators for the NHS: 1993: England: a consultation document*. London: Department of Health, 1993.
21. Department of Health. *On the State of the Public Health: the annual report of the Chief Medical Officer of the Department of Health for the year 1993*. London: HMSO, 1994; 117-8.

(b)   Primary health care

(i)   *Organisation of primary care*

The development of a primary-care-led NHS requires an understanding of the needs of individuals and of populations, to ensure that services are patient centred. The traditional skills of general practice need to be combined with a population-based perspective from public health medicine to make the best use of available NHS resources. As shown in the National Audit Office report *General practitioner fundholding in England*[1], published in December, GP fundholders have challenged traditional ways of providing care and now offer many novel services from their practice premises. There is a corresponding need to establish that such provision of services is effective and reaches those patients in greatest need. Alongside this major challenge, there must also to be clear public accountability, and publication of an accountability framework for GP fundholding is expected in mid-1995. GPs also need to be involved in the purchasing decisions of DHAs, and are ideally placed to know which services would most benefit their patients; health authorities need to build on their local knowledge to establish strong relations with GPs in this area.

133

Over 90% of GPs undertake health promotion programmes to identify and to reduce risk factors for coronary heart disease (CHD) and stroke. In addition, 90% of GPs run organised programmes of care for patients with diabetes mellitus and asthma (see page 140).

DH is working with the profession to reduce levels of bureaucracy for GPs and their staff, and a report on this subject is expected during 1995. Developments in information technology and the widespread use of computers by GPs have underpinned implementation of the LINK Programme, which connects practices electronically to Family Health Services Authorities (FHSAs) and enables some routine claims for payments to be made via computers without a need to complete paper returns. These developments should eventually reduce the administrative workload for GPs and their staff to a considerable extent.

Large GP rotas and co-operatives have continued to develop around the country as a means to provide emergency general medical services outside normal hours of work. Considerable interest continues to be expressed by GPs in the establishment of local groups to promote the delivery of high quality out-of-hours care by local doctors; ways to manage patient demand through telephone advice and emergency-surgery-based consultations, as well as maintaining an appropriate home-visiting service, are being increasingly explored.

The year saw a further increase in interest in the GP fundholding scheme in England. There are now nearly 1,700 such funds involving 8,760 GPs in 2,040 practices; they now cover 35% of the population. An extensive consultation exercise has shown that many GPs wish to take on even greater purchasing responsibilities on behalf of their patients, and many smaller practices are now interested in joining the fundholding scheme. The aim is to involve all GPs in purchasing decisions, and expansion of the scope of the scheme, together with the new community fundholding option from April 1996, will make many more practices eligible to join it in their own right.

Increasingly, GPs are developing more responsive services for local patients, sharing this development with local hospital consultants to make the best use of NHS resources. Examples across the country include:

-    a Trent initiative to establish additional weekend and evening sessions at the local hospital to improve access to care for all patients;

-    a North Tyneside medical centre's initiative to obtain a 24-hour laboratory service which has given increased cover to all local GP practices;

-    a Wakefield practice-based chiropodist service which provides care to patients of all local GPs;

-    Northumberland ophthalmology outreach clinics, which are shared by several local practices with support from a mobile ophthalmology unit;

-   Manchester GP fundholders who have bought endoscopy equipment to provide access to endoscopy services for all patients; *and*

-   joint appointment by a health commission and fundholders and a local social services department in the South and West RHA to employ a district nurse in the role of care manager to improve communication between primary and secondary care staff and to provide quicker assessment of elderly patients.

Other examples include improved quality of services in outpatients departments, pathology laboratory services and a reduction of duplicate radiograph investigations - all brought about by GPs and hospital staff sharing the agenda to improve local standards of care.

(ii)   Prescribing

GP fundholders have shown that prescribing costs can be contained without detriment to patient care, with their prescribing costs growing more slowly than those for other GPs. Around 500 non-fundholding GPs also participated successfully in prescribing incentive schemes which freed funding for other improved patient services. Benzodiazepine prescribing has fallen further while prescription of medication for asthma prophylaxis has continued to increase. Generic prescribing has increased from 44% in 1992/93 to 54% by the end of 1994. Nonetheless, the 9.9% real-terms increase of the primary care drugs bill in 1993/94, compared with the previous year (an 11.7% increase before allowing for inflation), points to the importance of cost-effectiveness in prescribing.

Prescribing information systems for GPs, DHAs and FHSAs have been greatly enhanced. Over 80% of GP practices, covering 90% of the population, are now computerised; standards for GP computing, including assessment of repeat prescribing and safety and price comparison systems, have been introduced and are annually reviewed. The Sowerby Unit's study on repeat prescribing showed that it made up 66% of items prescribed and 75% of total cost, and confirmed the value of regular reviews of individual patients to improve efficacy, safety and economy (Purves I, Kennedy J, unpublished data).

Two important reports related to prescribing were produced. The Audit Commission recommended increased prescribing for some conditions, such as asthma, while showing that significant savings compatible with maintained or enhanced quality of care were possible[2]. The Health Select Committee report commended the Department's prescribing initiatives and proposed further emphasis on information and support for doctors[3]. These reports are broadly welcomed by the Government and will inform future strategy on prescribing.

DH, in conjunction with the Association of the British Pharmaceutical Industry (ABPI), has developed guidelines for the economic evaluation of pharmaceuticals[4]. The Department is encouraging purchasers and prescribers to consider information about cost-effectiveness, and has provided guidance to purchasers on the development of policies for medicines provision that are coherent across primary and secondary care and take account of the views of health workers in all sectors.

Prescribing from a limited formulary by appropriately qualified nurses started on eight GP fundholding sites in October, and its effectiveness is to be fully evaluated.

(iii)   Professional development

Clinical audit and a relevant programme of continuing professional development are needed to achieve high quality primary health care. A growing understanding of the importance of close links between these two activities is reflected in the views of the Primary Health Care Working Group of COG, whose report will be published early in 1995. This report will set out possible further directions of provider development and quality assurance in primary care, and should be a helpful basis for local discussions.

The setting up of audit action groups (AAGs) has greatly facilitated audit in general practice; initially medical, these groups have extended their activities and now include representatives from other disciplines, management and lay people. A study has been commissioned to gain further information about these new activities, which include developmental work within practices and liaison with other agencies in different areas of work.

Provider development and clinical audit is seen to be the responsibility of the NHS at local level, but DH and the NHS Executive are investigating ways in which clinical audit and quality assurance in primary care can be securely developed.

(iv)   The way ahead

As the purchasing of secondary care and community services becomes increasingly led by GPs, a major challenge will be to secure the continued provision of good quality services within primary care itself. Whilst general practice has always been a broad church and should remain well differentiated, patients expect maintenance and improvement of standards as part of a natural progression of change and development. The development of a framework for primary care provision by professionals and managers in the NHS will still allow for diversification and development.

To fulfil these expectations, clinical audit and continuing professional education will require imaginative changes over several years, and will provide challenges for individual professionals, managers, and representatives of professional interest groups alike. However, the potential benefits for patients in terms of the delivery of a more integrated and holistic health care system will be substantial.

References

1.   National Audit Office. *General practitioner fundholding in England.* London: HMSO, 1994.

2. Audit Commission. *A prescription for improvement: towards more rational prescribing in general practice.* London: Audit Commission, 1994.
3. House of Commons. Health Committee. *Priority setting in the NHS: the NHS drugs budget: Session 1993-94.* London: HMSO, 1994. Chair: Ms Marion Roe.
4. Department of Health. *Virginia Bottomley welcomes pioneering guidelines for the economic evaluation of medicines.* London: Department of Health, 1994 (Press Release: H94/251).

(c)   Hospital services

(i)   Specialised services

In response to a report from the Clinical Standards Advisory Group (CSAG)[1], the arrangements for purchasing of highly specialised services were reviewed. The review concluded that there was a continued need for the Supra-Regional Services arrangements, and recommendations were made about the purchasing of other specialised services not meeting the current Supra-Regional criteria. There will now be a period of consultation on the report's recommendations.

(ii)   Cancer

Cancer continues to be a major concern to health care professionals and patients alike. There were about 145,000 deaths from cancer in England and Wales in 1989; cancers therefore represented the second most common cause of death after CHD[2]; and recent provisional figures indicate that they now cause more deaths than CHD. Some evidence of apparent variations in recorded outcome of cancer treatment within the UK is also a cause of public and professional concern[3].

In 1993, the Chief Medical Officers of England and Wales established an Expert Advisory Group on cancer, which prepared a report on the commissioning of cancer services as a consultation document in July 1994. The Group recommended three closely linked levels of cancer care: primary care, where cancer is usually first suspected and where much care, especially palliative care, is delivered; cancer units in most district general hospitals (DGHs), with specialist multidisciplinary teams to treat common cancers; and cancer centres within large general hospitals to treat the rarer cancers. Consultation has now ended and the revised report is being considered by Ministers.

The Standing Medical Advisory Committee (SMAC) has published a report on current good clinical practice in the management of lung cancer[4].

(iii)   Thromboprophylaxis

A conference on thromboprophylaxis, held in June at the Royal College of Surgeons of England and chaired by the Chief Medical Officer, has raised the profile of the subject further, building upon interest generated by recommendations by the National Confidential Enquiry into Peri-operative Deaths (NCEPOD)[5,6].

Thromboprophylaxis has been recognised as a priority for research by the Standing Group on Health Technology. A review of published research has been commissioned with a view to the production of clinical guidelines in the near future. The need for further research is also under review.

The NCEPOD report for 1992/93 should be published during 1995.

(iv)   Minimal access surgery

A notable feature of general surgical practice in recent years has been the rapid development of minimal access surgery (MAS). This change is part of a wider trend towards less invasive methods of diagnosis and treatment evident in many clinical specialties.

A wide variety of procedures may be classed as MAS. Some minimal access operations, such as arthroscopy and transurethral resection of the prostate (TURP) have been part of normal clinical practice for many years; others, such as laparoscopic surgery on the bowel or in the chest, are relatively new techniques and require further evaluation.

In 1994, the report of a Working Group chaired by Professor Cuschieri was issued by the Scottish Office Home and Health Department. This report made recommendations about clinical and management aspects of laparoscopic general surgery. In view of the importance of the subject, the Chief Medical Officer asked the SMAC to consider the report and provide further advice about MAS in the wider context of general surgical practice.

Four main aspects of MAS have already received special attention by the Department. In conjunction with the Wolfson Foundation it was agreed, early in 1992, to fund MAS training units, equipped with the most up-to-date audiovisual and simulator equipment. Two centres are now in action, based at the Royal College of Surgeons of England, in London, and at the General Infirmary, Leeds. These training units are developing links with other hospitals to extend further the range of training available. There is a third training unit in Scotland.

The Medical Devices Agency has set up an evaluation programme with particular emphasis on the contribution of televisual monitors, diathermy equipment and sterilisation. MAS has also been identified as a priority for central and NHS research funding. Reviews of published research have been commissioned and support is planned for further evaluation of the safety of MAS, including methods for the safe use of diathermy. DH has also supported Medical Research Council (MRC) projects on laparoscopic hernia and colorectal surgery; it funded major national audits of laparoscopic cholecystectomy and is reviewing other research proposals.

(v)   Osteoporosis

The Advisory Group on Osteoporosis, set up by Baroness Cumberlege, Parliamentary Under Secretary of State for Health in the House of Lords, to advise her on what was known about osteoporosis and on any need for further action, produced a draft report in May, which was then circulated for widespread consultation within the Department and the NHS; the results of this exercise were then considered by the Standing Medical Advisory Committee and the NHS Executive Board. Publication of the final report is expected early in 1995.

(vi)   Transplantation

Although about 2,700 transplants now take place every year the number waiting for such interventions continues to rise. The shortage of donor organs reflects increasing demand, as more patients are identified who might benefit from a transplant, and a fall in the main source of supply with the continued reduction in fatal road accidents. About one-third of potential donors are lost because relatives feel unable to give consent to organ removal. Research indicates that where a prior intention to donate organs in the event of death is known to relatives, few will refuse consent. Ministers therefore decided to establish a permanent computerised register which would hold a confidential record of people who wish to donate their organs, and which would be available for local transplant co-ordinators to check at any time.

The NHS Organ Donor Register was launched on 6 October. The Register is held at the UK Transplant Support Services Authority (UKTSSA) in Bristol alongside the national database of patients waiting for an organ transplant (see page 218). Donors are able to register when they apply for driving licences or by picking up the organ donor leaflet (ODR12R) containing a donor card and freepost registration form from main post offices, GP surgeries, libraries and other public places. Advertisements giving the freephone number 0800 555777 to obtain the ODR12Rs were displayed in national newspapers. Mr Tom Sackville MP, Parliamentary Under Secretary of State for Health in the House of Commons, sent a letter to all staff in the Department enclosing an ODR12R and inviting them to take this opportunity to record their own donor wishes, and also wrote to the editors of several hundred company newsletters. In December, a pilot scheme was set up in GP practices in Cheshire and the City and East London FHSAs to enable patients registering with a GP to record their donor wishes. By the end of 1994, nearly 150,000 people had applied to join the Register. A major publicity campaign for early 1995 was also planned.

References

1. Clinical Standards Advisory Group. *Access to and availability of specialist services: report of a CSAG Committee*. London: HMSO, 1993.
2. Office of Population Censuses and Surveys. *OPCS Annual Reference Volume 1989*. London: HMSO, 1994.
3. Thames Cancer Registry. *Cancer in South East England 1990*. Sutton (Surrey): Thames Cancer Registry, 1991.
4. Standing Medical Advisory Committee. *Management of lung cancer: current clinical practices: report of a working group*. London: Department of Health, 1994. Chair: Professor Michael Whitehouse.
5. Campling GA, Devlin HB, Hoite RW, et al. *The report of the National Confidential Enquiry into Peri-operative Deaths: 1991/92*. London: National Confidential Enquiry into Peri-operative Deaths, 1993.
6. Department of Health. *On the State of the Public Health: the annual report of the Chief Medical Officer of the Department of Health for the year 1993*. London: HMSO, 1994; 123.

(d)   Diabetes mellitus

In August, the Clinical Standards Advisory Group reported on standards of clinical care for people with diabetes mellitus[1]. DH accepted the need to encourage purchasers to ensure adequate local services for patients with diabetes mellitus, with appropriate standards specified in contracts. A series of epidemiologically based needs assessment reviews, including one on diabetes mellitus[2], was published to help health authorities to assess health care needs.

Also in March, Mr Tom Sackville MP, Parliamentary Under Secretary of State for Health in the House of Commons, addressed a DH-funded conference at the Royal College of Physicians. The aim was to exchange information on the work of the joint DH/British Diabetic Association Task Force for diabetes mellitus. The Task Force made its second report in November; DH is considering how best to develop purchaser guidance, initially in three target areas - blindness, renal complications and foot complications.

References

1. Clinical Standards Advisory Group. *Clinical Standards Advisory Group report on diabetes mellitus.* London: Department of Health, 1994.
2. Stevens A, Raftery J, eds. *Health care needs assessment: the epidemiologically based needs assessment reviews (vols I & II).* Oxford: Radcliffe Press, 1994.

(e)   Asthma

In October, Ministers announced a conference on asthma, to be organised by DH and the Department of the Environment (DoE) in association with the Institute for Environment and Health (IEH) and the National Asthma Campaign. This one-day conference, to be held in Autumn 1995, will focus on the causes of asthma and what everyone can do to alleviate its effects and to help to prevent new cases. A wide range of interested parties, including patient groups, will be represented.

It is estimated that there are some 1,500 new cases of occupational asthma in the UK annually[1]. In April, the Health and Safety Executive (HSE) launched its 'Breathe Freely' campaign to raise awareness of occupational asthma and thereby reduce its incidence. The campaign reminds employers of their responsibilities to control exposure to inhaled materials which can cause asthma.

In recognition of professional and public concern about a possible link between air pollution and asthma, DH asked the Committee on the Medical Effects of Air Pollutants (COMEAP) for advice: a sub-group was set up to examine the relevant evidence, and a report is expected to be published in late 1995.

Many people with asthma use aerosol inhalers to deliver medication directly to the lungs; these contain a chlorinated fluorocarbon (CFC) propellant. Under EC Regulation 3952/92, production of CFCs for use in non-essential products was scheduled to be phased out by 1 January 1995. However, an exemption was agreed for asthma inhalers to allow time for the development of alternative propellants to ensure continuity of inhaler supply.

Reference

1.   Newman Taylor A. Environmental determinants of asthma. *Lancet* (in press).

(f)   Complementary medicine

Based on the model of the Osteopathy Act 1993[1], a Private Members Bill to regulate chiropractors, introduced by Mr David Lidington MP, received Royal Assent in July[2]. The Chiropractors Act 1994[2] provides for the establishment of a General Chiropractic Council which will develop, promote and regulate the profession of chiropractic. The Council will ensure that only those persons who are suitably qualified both personally and professionally, and who are registered under the statutory scheme, are allowed to practise as and call themselves chiropractors. Work is now in hand to establish the General Chiropractic Council and its education, investigating, professional conduct and health committees.

Following the successful passage of the Osteopathy and Chiropractors Acts, interest in statutory regulation has been shown by other groups of complementary therapists, such as practitioners of acupuncture and homoeopathy. Statutory regulation is primarily a matter for the professional groups themselves to pursue. Any move towards statutory regulation would require the broad support of the practitioners concerned, be founded on a successful system of voluntary registration which embraces an appropriate and enforceable code of practice, and have the support of medical and scientific evidence and opinion.

References

1.   *Osteopathy Act 1993.* London: HMSO, 1993.
2.   *Chiropractors Act 1994.* London: HMSO, 1994.

(g)   Mental health

(i)   Mental health and primary care

Most mental illness is treated in a primary care rather than a secondary care setting. Depression and anxiety are the most common conditions; long-term severe mental illness is much less common, but very disabling. A number of DH-funded projects to optimise the primary care of mental illness are now nearing completion[1,2].

A joint venture between DH, the Royal College of General Practitioners (RCGP) and the Gatsby Charitable Foundation has set up a national network of regional GP mental health fellows to advise primary health care teams. A study of GP facilitators for mental health has been completed and results will be available shortly. The Exeter depression audit package is being developed and work in Bath is evaluating GP-based models of care for depression, anxiety and alcohol misuse, and the contribution of primary care to the management of schizophrenia.

DH continues to provide financial and technical support to the professional and public education initiatives of the 'Defeat Depression' campaign organised by the RCGP and the Royal College of Psychiatrists. Through its research and development programme, the Department also funds various projects to assess and to improve the primary care of mental illness.

(ii)   Occupational mental health

In January, DH convened the Mental Health at Work Inter-Agency Group to co-ordinate strategies for occupational mental health. It comprises other Government Departments, relevant advisory bodies, and organisations representing employers and employees. The *ABC of mental health in the workplace*, a resource pack for medium and small businesses endorsed by the group, was launched by the Secretary of State for Health in November[3]. The pack provides key facts on mental health, methods to prevent and to tackle mental health problems, and references to further information.

The Department held 'Mental health at work' information stands at the Confederation of British Industry (CBI) conference and at the Royal Agricultural Show, where the issue of rural stress was highlighted. DH emphasised its own commitment to action by issuing a staff mental health policy in 1994. The mental health of the NHS workforce remains an NHS research and development priority and a longitudinal study of influences that affect health care professionals continued, as did Departmental support for the 'Health at Work in the NHS' project.

(iii)   Confidential Inquiry into Homicides and Suicides

An independent Confidential Inquiry was established by Ministers in 1991 "to inquire into ... homicides or suicides by people under the care of, or recently discharged from the specialist psychiatric service; ... and to recommend measures designed to reduce the number of such incidents". The Inquiry published an interim report on homicides in August[4].

Some 450-500 people are convicted of homicide annually in England and Wales; between July 1992 and December 1993, the inquiry identified only 34 instances in which the perpetrator had been in contact with the specialist psychiatric service in the previous 12 months. The report described the 22 such cases where data collection was complete. Of the perpetrators, 68% were male (of whom 73% had schizophrenia), whereas, of the women, 71% had affective disorder. Only two victims were strangers to the assailant. In 59% of cases, some failure of compliance with the treatment plan had preceded the incident. The Inquiry recommended, among other suggestions, more effective application of the care programme approach[5] to improve continuity of care. While emphasising that homicides by mentally ill people were very rare, DH welcomed the report and the Inquiry's support for initiatives to ensure safe and effective community care, such as supervision registers[6] and the proposed new powers for supervised discharge.

(iv)　　*Services for people with severe mental illness*

The second edition of the Health of the Nation Key Area Handbook on mental illness[7] set out a practical framework to establish the range of services required to assess and to meet the needs of people with severe mental illness. The development of comprehensive mental health services was studied in a number of national reviews[8,9,10,11], which highlighted the need to provide services for the severely mentally ill and to develop a balanced range of hospital and community provision. Supervision registers were introduced to ensure that services focused on the most vulnerable.

The Mental Health Task Force London project was commissioned to examine services in twelve London health districts. A team of practising managers and clinicians, with representatives of user and carer organisations, met with local purchasers and providers to identify their difficulties and to formulate action plans. Priorities included more active implementation of the care programme approach and supervision registers; strategies to address the pressure on acute beds; the need to develop non-acute, 24-hour staffed community and hospital places; enhanced inter-Agency working; and the development of responsive services for people from different ethnic and cultural backgrounds. A follow-up review showed that many DHAs were progressing well with their action plans.

DH has had a particular focus on those with severe mental illness in different ethnic and cultural groups. Initiatives have included training and dissemination of information, collaborative ventures with the Royal College of Psychiatrists, joint funding of a GP senior fellow in mental health, the 'Defeat Depression' campaign, publication of an educational booklet for black users and carers, and a jointly funded conference and post on ethnicity, culture and mental illness.

The OPCS National Psychiatric Morbidity Survey was completed and its findings should start to be published early in 1995. During next year a series of reports should be published to inform local needs assessments and the development of mental health services. Field trials of the Health of the Nation Outcome Scale (HoNOS) were completed and progress is being made to incorporate this simple yardstick of mental health into the development of a new system for routine data collection[12].

Additional initiatives to assist the development of services have included production of training and audit programmes on the role of the key worker and the implementation of the care programme approach, regional purchaser development programmes, provider management education and support through the King's Fund, and commissioning of a study on schizophrenia by the Clinical Standards Advisory Group. The importance of social care through housing and financial support to clinical outcomes has recently been highlighted. A series of joint Department of the Environment/DH seminars on housing the mentally ill have been organised.

Guidance was published on the discharge of mentally disordered people from hospital[13]; it aims to ensure that patients are discharged only when and if they are ready to leave hospital, that any risk is minimal and managed effectively, and that patients when discharged get the support and supervision which they need.

(v)   Services for mentally disordered offenders

An expert Working Group reported on the provision of high security psychiatric services for patients in England and Wales, and recommended radical changes to funding and management arrangements[14]. Ministers commissioned further work from officials to advise them by January 1995 on whether the report's recommendations were compatible with their obligations to maintain the security and quality of such services and to ensure value for money. Decisions would be taken in the light of this further advice.

A second Working Group reported to the Home Office and DH on the treatment and management of people with psychopathic disorder[15]. The report concluded that there was insufficient information to determine whether people suffering from psychopathic disorder could be successfully treated. It also made recommendations regarding new legal provisions, research and service provision. Comments received during a consultation period are under review by the two Departments.

Increased numbers of patients continue to transfer from prison to NHS health care under the provisions of the Mental Health Act 1983[16]. 746 prisoners transferred in 1994, of whom 234 had been sentenced and 512 were on remand. The reasons for this very considerable increase from 103 transfers in 1982 to the present level are unclear, but may include better detection of mental disorder at all points of contact between mentally disordered people and the criminal justice system, greater access to facilities in the NHS and closer co-operation between the NHS and the prison service.

Partly as a result of this rise in transfers from prison, there has been considerable pressure on beds offering treatment in conditions of medium security. Over £45 million of central capital funding have been provided between 1991 and 1995 to develop medium secure beds; in 1994, an additional £4.4 million were made available. There are now over 750 purpose-built medium secure places in the NHS, some 500 other NHS secure beds and 450 secure beds in the independent sector. Most of these services were originally intended to provide care for up to two years, but a survey has shown that over one-quarter of the beds were occupied by patients needing longer term inpatient care. The need was often for longer term care at a level of security below that in medium secure units, but greater than that commonly available in the general psychiatric service. Responding to this need, which was also identified in the second national needs assessment exercise[17], many services are now developing specialist facilities to offer care at this lower level of security.

Improved training, particularly inter-Agency training, for those working with mentally disordered offenders was identifed as an important need in the original Reed reviews[18]. A training pack[19] for social workers was commissioned from the National Association for the Care and Resettlement of Offenders (NACRO) and launched with a series of seven conferences.

(vi)   Mental health legislation

In February, the Court of Appeal in the case of *R v Mental Health Review Tribunal ex parte A*[20] held that for the purposes of the Mental Health Act 1983[16] a patient is not untreatable simply because he or she refuses to accept the treatment being offered. In this particular case the treatment was psychotherapy in a group setting, but the Court stressed the very wide definition of medical treatment under the Act which includes nursing, and also "care, habilitation and rehabilitation under medical supervision".

A consultation paper issued by the Department in October sought views on promoting the use of guardianship under the Mental Health Act 1983[16] or extending its powers, but suggested that any such initiative should be considered in the light of experience of the proposed new power of supervised discharge.

Supervised discharge was initially proposed in 1993[21]. Following widespread consultation on the proposal a Mental Health Bill was announced in the Queen's Speech in November. Supervised discharge will address the problem of so-called 'revolving door' patients by requiring them to abide by the terms of a care plan drawn up before they leave hospital; failure to comply would lead to an immediate review of the case and possible readmission to hospital. The Bill will also seek to extend the maximum period of leave of absence for detained patients from the current six months to one year, and correct the anomaly by which the power to return detained patients who go absent without leave lapses after 28 days.

References

1. Jenkins R. Developments in the primary care of mental illness: a forward look. *Int Rev Psychiatry* 1992; **4:** 237-42.
2. Lloyd K, Jenkins R, The economics of depression in primary care: Department of Health initiatives. *Br J Psychiatry* (in press).
3. Department of Health. *ABC of mental health in the workplace.* London: Department of Health, 1994.
4. Steering Committee of the Confidential Inquiry into Homicides and Suicides by Mentally Ill People. *A preliminary report on homicide.* London: Confidential Inquiry into Homicides and Suicides by Mentally Ill People, 1994.
5. Department of Health. *The care programme approach for people with a mental illness referred to the specialist psychiatric service.* Heywood (Lancashire): Department of Health, 1990 (Health Circular: HC(90)23, Local Authority Social Services Letter: LASSL(90)11).
6. Department of Health. *Introduction of supervision registers for mentally ill people from 1 April 1994.* Heywood (Lancashire): Department of Health, 1994 (Health Service Guidelines: HSG(94)5).
7. Department of Health. *The Health of the Nation Key Area Handbook: mental illness. 2nd edn.* London: HMSO, 1994.
8. Audit Commission. *Finding a place: a review of mental health services for adults.* London: HMSO, 1994.
9. Mental Health Foundation. *Creating community care: report of the Mental Health Foundation into community care for people with severe mental illness.* London: Mental Health Foundation, 1994. Chair: Sir William Utting.
10. Ritchie J, Dick D, Lingham R. *The Report of the Inquiry into the Care and Treatment of Christopher Clunis.* London: HMSO, 1994.

11. House of Commons. Health Committee. *Better off in the community? The care of people who are seriously mentally ill: first report by the Health Committee: Session 1993-94.* London: HMSO, 1994 (HC 102; vol I).
12. Department of Health. HoNOS: a psychiatric thermometer. *CMO's Update* 1994; **4:** 7.
13. Department of Health. *Guidance on the discharge of mentally disordered people and their continuing care in the community.* London: Department of Health, 1994 (Health Service Guidelines: HSG(94)27).
14. Department of Health. *Report of the Working Group on High Security and Related Psychiatric Provision.* London: Department of Health, 1994. Chair: Dr John Reed.
15. Department of Health, Home Office. *Report of the Department of Health and Home Office Working Group on Psychopathic Disorder.* London: Department of Health, 1994. Chair: Dr John Reed.
16. *Mental Health Act 1983.* London: HMSO, 1983.
17. Department of Health. *On the State of the Public Health 1993: the annual report of the Chief Medical Officer of the Department of Health for the year 1993.* London: HMSO, 1994; 127-9.
18. Department of Health, Home Office. *Review of health and social services for mentally disordered offenders and others requiring similar services: final summary report.* London. HMSO, 1992 (Cm. 2088). Chair: Dr John Reed.
19. National Association for the Care and Resettlement of Offenders. *Working with mentally disordered offenders: a training pack for social services staff and others dealing with mentally disordered offenders.* London: Department of Health, 1994.
20. *R v Mental Health Review Tribunal ex parte A.* QB Cos 93-1099-D (1994).
21. Department of Health. *Legal powers on the care of mentally ill people in the community: report of the internal review.* London: Department of Health, 1993. Chairs: Miss Dora Pease, Dr John Reed.

(h)   Maternity and child health services

(i)   Implementation of 'Changing Childbirth'

The Report for 1993[1] mentioned that consultation on the Expert Maternity Group's Report, *Changing Childbirth*[2], was in progress as the year ended. Wide acceptance of its recommendations, which were based on the principle of woman-centred care, led to a Government decision to promulgate them within the NHS[3]. In February, the Royal College of Obstetricians and Gynaecologists (RCOG) held a study group attended by representatives of other professional bodies involved in maternity care to consider the implications in depth; its conclusions[4] were in line with those of the Expert Maternity Group.

DH appointed an implementation team to promote the changes and an advisory group to advise on educational and training aspects. Around £350,000 were allocated to support a range of pilot implementation projects, and videotapes giving information about choices were commissioned. In April, the Department published a Patient's Charter leaflet[5] for maternity services. The RCOG stepped up its development of a standard maternity record, which could be extremely valuable in the changing service.

Work began within DH on ways to monitor change by the ten indicators of successful implementation listed in the Expert Maternity Group's report. An evaluation study of new midwifery practice was also commissioned from the National Perinatal Epidemiology Unit.

(ii)   Confidential Enquiries into Maternal Deaths

The report on *Confidential Enquiries into Maternal Deaths in the United Kingdom 1988-1990* was published in January[6]. From this report - which is the latest of a series which began in England and Wales in 1952 and is the second to cover the UK as a whole - a maternal mortality rate of 10 per 100,000 maternities has been derived.

The three main causes of deaths directly related to obstetric complications of pregnancy, labour and the puerperium have remained the same since the 1985-1987 report: thrombosis and thrombo-embolism, hypertensive disorders of pregnancy and haemorrhage. The numbers of deaths in the first two categories have remained constant since the previous triennium, whereas deaths due to haemorrhage have doubled. Deaths directly due to anaesthesia continued to decline.

The report included illustrative case histories and identified elements of substandard care, which related not only to clinical care and support facilities but also to patient behaviour beyond the influence of clinicians. It also included a review of data collection systems and definitions of maternal deaths used in European countries. Under-reporting of maternal death is a common feature throughout Europe, and international comparisons were shown to be unreliable.

The report's recommendations, intended to improve maternity service provision in consultant maternity units, emphasised the need for progress in the following areas: deficiencies in staffing structure, blood availability, high-dependency care facilities and the establishment of protocols for the management of life-threatening conditions. Attention was also drawn to the need for greater awareness of thrombo-embolic disorders, for improved initial and continuing training for maternity unit staff and for improved counselling of women with potential life-threatening conditions.

DH has encouraged implementation of the recommendations of the report via a letter from the Chief Medical Officer to purchasers and providers of maternity services[7], *CMO's Update*[8] and in an Executive Letter[9]. An audit of the outcome of recommendations of previous Reports was published separately in *Health Trends*[10]. Deficiencies in the availability of recommended facilities in the UK were highlighted: for example, more than one in ten consultant units did not have a 24-hour blood bank facility on site, and one in four did not have an intensive care unit.

(iii)   *Folic acid and prevention of neural tube defects*

In 1994, the first Product Licence for a 400 microgram folic acid supplement was granted and more food supplements became available. The Medicines (Advertising) Regulations 1994[11] permitted licensed products to be advertised for the prevention of neural tube defects, including spina bifida. A major educational programme is planned to start in 1995.

(iv)   *Human Fertilisation and Embryology Authority*

The licensing work of the Human Fertilisation and Embryology Authority (HFEA) has continued in a highly effective manner[12]. In 1994, the first licences were issued for intracytoplasmic sperm injection. This procedure[13], in which a single sperm is injected into an egg to effect fertilisation, has been recognised as a major advance in attempts to treat male infertility.

In January, the HFEA issued a public consultation document[14] on the use of donated ovarian tissue in embryo research and assisted conception. A key feature of the resulting report[15] was the conclusion that eggs derived from foetuses are not acceptable for infertility treatment: such use will be prohibited by the Criminal Justice and Public Order Act 1994[16]. The Authority also began work on a consultation document about the publication of treatment success rates, which will be issued early in 1995.

(v)   Sudden infant death syndrome

The Report for 1993 recorded that preliminary data on the incidence of sudden infant death syndrome (SIDS) indicated that the low level recorded in 1992 had been maintained[17]. This finding was confirmed, with a fall to 0.7 per 1,000 live births in 1993[18]. There has been a fall of more than 70% in SIDS mortality between 1988 and 1993.

In 1990, the Chief Medical Officer set up an expert working group to investigate the hypothesis by Mr P R Mitchell and Mr B A Richardson that SIDS might be caused by the microbial generation of phosphine, stibine or arsine from compounds present in the polyvinylchloride (PVC) used in some cot mattresses and their covers. The report of the group (the Turner Report), which was published in 1991, concluded that this hypothesis was not supported by experimental evidence[19]. During 1994, two Independent Television (ITV) programmes challenged these findings. However, the Chief Medical Officer received advice that the programmes provided no evidence to invalidate the Turner Report; that research reported in the ITV programmes was limited and inadequate; and that further information would be needed before a consistent assessment could be made[20].

The Chief Medical Officer set up an expert group, chaired by Lady Limerick, to review earlier findings and any new evidence, looking particularly at the postulated causal relations between chemicals and cot deaths[21].

(vi)   Prophylaxis of vitamin K deficiency bleeding in infants

Last year's Report[22] drew attention to a number of new studies into the reported carcinogenic effects of vitamin K.

In July, the Chief Medical Officer met representatives of medical and nursing professional bodies to discuss current issues on the administration of vitamin K. Concerns raised included the propriety of administering vitamin K by mouth when it was unlicensed for this route; the likely delay before a licensed oral vitamin K preparation would be available; variations in clinical policy and practice, and in the provision of guidance and local protocols; the possible increased risk of bleeding in some children given vitamin K orally, compared with intramuscular administration; and concerns about the consistency of practice in giving timely information to parents to enable them to give informed consent.

The meeting agreed that advice setting out good practice could best be prepared by the relevant professions. This advice should set out: the basis for vitamin K prophylaxis; the status of existing research findings and impending studies; the importance of early identification and referral of children at risk of vitamin K deficiency bleeding; and the need for agreed and known local policies and practice, including the content and availability of information for parents. After further consideration of research in progress, the preparation of guidelines was deferred to take into account the results of that research, which are now expected to be published during 1995.

(vii) *Retinopathy of prematurity*

Over the last 40 years, the survival rate for babies with a birthweight of less than 1,000 grams has increased from 4% to 66%; survival of those with a birthweight between 1,000 grams and 1,500 grams has risen from 38% to 80%. With this improved survival, the incidence of retinopathy of prematurity (ROP) has also increased. Both the incidence and severity of acute ROP rise with decreasing maturity, and about 50% of babies with a birthweight below 1,500 grams develop some degree of retinopathy. Severe disease is confined mainly to infants of less than 1,500 grams birthweight or less than 31 weeks' gestation, among whom the incidence of severe (stage 3 or 4) disease is about 10%[23].

Until recently, there was no means to prevent or to treat ROP, but reports from the Multicentre Trial of Cryotherapy for ROP now indicate that the unfavourable outcome of stage 3 disease can be significantly improved by treatment[23], and have raised the issue of screening for this condition. DH has therefore sought the views of professional bodies on proposals to evaluate these findings in practice, with an aim to reduce the incidence of severe visual impairment in children at high risk of ROP. These bodies agreed the need for a study to determine the pattern of screening and treatment policies and practice in the NHS and their relation to locally available resources, and to obtain data on outcomes in infants screened or treated for ROP, with attention to questions of cost-effectiveness and quality of care.

The Department has now commissioned a nationwide research, training and audit programme with the collaboration of the Royal College of Ophthalmologists, the British Association of Perinatal Medicine, and the British Paediatric Association. This programme will begin early in 1995 with a survey of the incidence of babies with severe ROP, and of current screening, treatment and counselling practices undertaken by paediatricians and ophthalmologists in the UK. This will be complemented by a training programme to be funded by DH as part of the Minimal Access Therapy Training Unit. During 1997-98 there will be a follow-up study of all babies with stage 3 ROP. The last part of the programme, in late 1998, will be a repeat survey to determine and to quantify changes in screening, treatment and counselling practice.

(viii)   Paediatric intensive care

Last year's Report[24] recorded the publication of *The care of critically ill children*[25], the report of a multidisciplinary working party on paediatric intensive care. The NHS Executive commissioned a review by the NHS Centre for Reviews and Dissemination (CRD) to complement the report[26]. This review looked at the weight of evidence available to support the conclusions and recommendations of the report, and drew attention to deficiencies in the information available for the UK in regard to the numbers of critically ill children, measures of illness severity, the content of care, and outcomes; it also pointed to the small amount of relevant health services research that had been published. The report, the review and observations of international groups revealed a diversity of opinion on the required level of provision of services, the optimum size of units and their disposition, and their patterns of staffing, but did help to identify areas where there is a lack of research evidence. The differences of opinion did not extend to the clinical or pastoral needs of very sick children and their families.

Some of the research needed is being incorporated in the NHS research and development programme. The results should allow a more informed discussion about the factors which influence the survival of critically ill children. Work planned includes the development of casemix and outcome measures; the identification of ways to determine the impact of qualitative and organisational aspects of intensive care; and ways to ensure increased accuracy of cost estimation. Alongside the subjects of this CRD review, work has begun into the implications of developments in paediatric intensive care for postgraduate medical education and for children's nurses and their training.

Lastly, fulfilling a commitment made by the then Minister of Health in 1993, DHAs were asked to review and report on their needs for paediatric intensive care[27].

(ix)   Confidential Enquiry into Stillbirths and Deaths in Infancy

The first year of data collection for the Confidential Enquiry into Stillbirths and Deaths in Infancy (CESDI) was 1993[28]. During 1994, the CESDI programme comprised: collection of information on all deaths between 20 weeks gestation and one year-of-age; confidential enquiries on intrapartum-related deaths in normally formed babies aged up to 4 completed weeks and with birthweights of 1.5 kg and above; continuation of the case-control studies and confidential enquiries into sudden unexpected deaths in infancy (SUDI); pilot work on a case-control study of antepartum stillbirths; an audit of necropsy reports on CESDI cases; completion of the report on a comparative study of CESDI assessment panels; an evaluation study of CESDI methods; production of the CESDI newsletter; and the provision of workshops for CESDI co-ordinators. Information for bereaved parents on post-mortem investigations was translated into nine languages and distributed in January.

The reduction from 14 to 8 in the number of NHS Regions on 1 April, and computing changes at OPCS, caused minimal disruption to the programme although receipt and analysis of reports was delayed: the National Advisory Body's (NAB's) Annual Report for 1993 was prepared for publication early in 1995. Of the 9,221 deaths reported for 1993, 388 were included in the intrapartum-related confidential enquiries and 128 were included in the SUDI study. On the basis of the confidential enquiry results, the NAB (chaired by Lady Littler), identified a number of potentially avoidable factors and considered the recommendations it might make in relation to risk management, communication skills, training, and guidelines for clinical management, including those relating to resuscitation of newborn babies.

The NAB decided to continue the main components of the CESDI programme for 1995, with no change to the criteria for confidential enquiries on intrapartum-related deaths. SUDI investigations, with a modified protocol and questionnaire, will be conducted in three new NHS Regions, thereby including two more of the former NHS Regions; these investigations will include more detail in relation to postulated risk factors. Antepartum stillbirth studies will be conducted in two new NHS Regions and the programme will also incorporate follow-up of the pathology audit and the study of assessment panels. The rapid reporting form for all deaths will include ethnic group, using the OPCS classification, and all terminations of pregnancy under the Abortion Act 1967[29,30,31] at 20 or more weeks of gestation.

(x)   Congenital malformations

The great majority of babies are normal at birth, but some (about 1-2%) are found to be imperfectly formed in some way. During 1994, there were sporadic reports of apparently unusual occurrences of a number of congenital anomalies, which included anomalies of the eye (anophthalmia and microphthalmia) and of the limbs. These reports again drew attention to the distress of parents of affected children and the anxieties of prospective parents, and raised much public and Parliamentary concern. The reports also generated considerable speculation on possible causes, especially environmental ones.

Microphthalmia and anophthalmia

In 1993, alleged clusters of microphthalmia/anophthalmia in England and Wales were suggested by the media to be linked to exposure to the pesticide benomyl. Ministers asked for the available data to be reviewed and undertook to commission additional necessary research[32]. Preliminary assessment of the reports concluded that the evidence was insufficient to point to clustering, mainly because of the lack of exact diagnostic information and the want of evidence for a link with benomyl. DH has commissioned a study to compile and validate a register of all cases of anophthalmia in infants born in Great Britain during the period 1987-92; this register will provide a sound basis for assessment of urban/rural differences and the geographical distribution of affected children. The results of this study are expected to be available in 1997.

Limb reduction defects

There have also been sporadic reports of alleged clusters of congenital limb defects. Most of these reports were from coastal areas, leading to speculation on possible environmental factors. However, studies in this country and abroad found no coastal bias: these included studies using data for England and Wales collected through the OPCS Congenital Malformations Notification Scheme, and a more detailed study from the Northern RHA in England[33,34,35,36]. These findings did not wholly satisfy public concerns and DH set up an Expert Group to advise the director of NHS research and development whether useful new information could be gained from further research. Its report will be published early in 1995.

(xi)   Gene Therapy Advisory Committee

The Report for 1993[37] recorded the establishment of the Gene Therapy Advisory Committee (GTAC), chaired by Professor Dame June Lloyd. GTAC met for the first time in November 1993, and held a further five meetings during 1994. Its first report to Ministers is due to be published early in 1995.

By December 1994, GTAC (and its predecessor the Committee on the Ethics of Gene Therapy) had received 12 proposals for gene therapy research in human subjects. Ten were approved in principle for studies in the following diseases: severe combined immunodeficiency (1), cystic fibrosis (4), malignant melanoma (2), lymphoma (2) and neuroblastoma (1). Protocols have also been submitted for studies in breast cancer and acute myeloid leukaemia.

GTAC set as one of its very first priorities the preparation of guidance for researchers. Much had been learnt from the work of the Recombinant DNA Advisory Committee (RAC) in the United States of America. Their experience, together with that gained with the first proposals seen by GTAC and its Secretariat, and discussions with UK medical scientists, all contributed to the development of the GTAC guidelines which were published in September[38]. These guidelines emphasise key aspects of information which are common to all areas of gene therapy research and are essential to enable the Committee to make an adequate assessment of the ethical acceptability of the protocol, taking into account its scientific merit and potential benefits.

The Committee's approach to the review of protocols is intended to be both detailed and challenging, so as to maintain public confidence in the system of review. But the review process should also enable sound research to proceed and to move towards therapeutic applications.

(xii)   Code of practice on special educational needs and circulars on 'Pupils with problems'

In September, the Department for Education (DFE) and the Welsh Office published a Code of Practice on the identification and assessment of special educational needs[39], as required by the Education Act 1993[40]. The Code highlights the need for close inter-agency co-operation in the identification and assessment of special educational needs, with sections devoted to the involvement of child health services and social services: in particular, there is guidance on the role of the designated medical officer for special educational needs.

In May, DH and DFE collaborated on the production of a set of circulars, collectively entitled 'Pupils with problems'. These included three joint DFE/DH circulars concerning the education of children with emotional and behavioural difficulties[41]; the education of sick children[42]; and the education of children being looked after by local authorities[43].

References

1. Department of Health. *On the State of the Public Health: the annual report of the Chief Medical Officer of the Department of Health for the year 1993.* London: HMSO, 1994; 130-1.
2. Department of Health. *Changing Childbirth: part 1: report of the Expert Maternity Group.* London: HMSO, 1993. Chair: Baroness Cumberlege.
3. Department of Health. *Woman-centred maternity services.* Heywood (Lancashire): Department of Health, 1994 (Executive Letter: EL(94)9).
4. Chamberlain GVA, Patel N, eds. *The future of the maternity services.* London: Royal College of Obstetricians and Gynaecologists, 1994.
5. Department of Health. *The Patient's Charter for maternity services.* London: Department of Health, 1994.
6. Department of Health, Welsh Office, Scottish Office Home and Health Department, Northern Ireland Department of Health and Social Services. *Report on Confidential Enquiries into Maternal Deaths in the United Kingdom 1988-1990.* London: HMSO, 1994.
7. Department of Health. *Report on Confidential Enquiries into Maternal Deaths in the United Kingdom 1988-1990.* Heywood (Lancashire): Department of Health, 1994 (Professional Letter: PL/CMO(94)1).
8. Department of Health. Maternal deaths. *CMO's Update* 1994; **2**: 6.
9. Department of Health. *Improving the effectiveness of the NHS.* Heywood (Lancashire): Department of Health, 1994 (Executive Letter: EL(94)74).
10. Hibbard B, Milner D. Reports on Confidential Enquiries into Maternal Deaths: an audit of previous recommendations. *Health Trends* 1994; **26**: 26-8.
11. *Medicines (Advertising) Regulations 1994.* London: HMSO, 1994 (Statutory Instrument: SI 1994 no. 1932).
12. Human Fertilisation and Embryology Authority. *Third annual report.* London: Human Fertilisation and Embryology Authority, 1994.
13. Van Steirteghem AL, Liu J, Joris H, et al. Higher success rate by intracytoplasmic sperm injection than by subzonal insemination: report of a second series of 300 consecutive treatment cycles. *Hum Reprod* 1993; **8**: 1055-60.
14. Human Fertilisation and Embryology Authority. *Donated ovarian tissue in embryo research and assisted conception: public consultation document.* London: Human Fertilisation and Embryology Authority, 1994.
15. Human Fertilisation and Embryology Authority. *Donated ovarian tissue in embryo research and assisted conception - a report.* London: Human Fertilisation and Embryology Authority, 1994.
16. *Criminal Justice and Public Order Act 1994.* London: HMSO, 1994.
17. Department of Health. *On the State of the Public Health: the annual report of the Chief Medical Officer of the Department of Health for the year 1993.* London: HMSO, 1994; 132.
18. Office of Population Censuses and Surveys. *Sudden infant deaths 1989-93.* London: Office of Population Censuses and Surveys, 1994 (Monitor series: DH3 94/1).
19. Department of Health. *Sudden infant death syndrome (SIDS): report of the Expert Working Group inquiring into the hypothesis that toxic gases evolved from chemicals in cot mattress covers and cot mattresses are a cause of SIDS.* London: HMSO, 1991. Chair: Professor Paul Turner.
20. Department of Health. *Government statement on 'The Cook Report' cot deaths programme.* London: Department of Health, 1994 (Press Release: H94/528).
21. Department of Health. *Expert Group to investigate cot death theories.* London: Department of Health, 1994 (Press Release: H94/553).
22. Department of Health. *On the State of the Public Health: the annual report of the Chief Medical Officer of the Department of Health for the year 1993.* London: HMSO, 1994; 132-3.
23. Fielder AR, Levene MI. Screening for retinopathy of prematurity. *Arch Dis Childh* 1992; **67**: 860-7.
24. Department of Health. *On the State of the Public Health: the annual report of the Chief Medical Officer of the Department of Health for the year 1993.* London: HMSO, 1994; 134.
25. Fleming P, Matthew D. *The care of critically ill children: report of the Multidisciplinary Working Party of Paediatric Intensive Care convened by the British Paediatric Association.* London: British Paediatric Association, 1993.

153

26. NHS Centre for Reviews and Dissemination. *Which way forward for the care of critically ill children?* York: NHS Centre for Reviews and Dissemination (University of York), 1994.
27. Department of Health. *Paediatric intensive care.* Heywood (Lancashire): Department of Health, 1994 (Executive Letter: EL(94)10).
28. Department of Health. *On the State of the Public Health: the annual report of the Chief Medical Officer of the Department of Health for the year 1993.* London: HMSO, 1994; 134-5.
29. *Abortion Act 1967.* London: HMSO, 1967.
30. *Abortion Act 1967 (as amended by Statutory Instrument: SI 480c.10).* London: HMSO, 1991.
31. *The Human Fertilisation and Embryology Act 1990 (Commencement no. 2 and Transitional Provision) Order 1991.* London: HMSO, 1991 (Statutory Instrument: SI 1991 no. 480).
32. House of Commons. Parliamentary Debate. Children born without eyes. *Hansard* 25 March 1993: Col 432-3.
33. Botting B. Limb reduction defects and coastal areas. *Lancet* 1994; **343**: 1033-4.
34. Castella EE, da Graca Dura M. Limb reduction defects. *Lancet* 1994; **343**: 1034.
35. Mastrolacova P. Limb reduction defects. *Lancet* 1994; **343**: 1034-5.
36. Wright MJ, Newell JN, Charlton ME, Hey EN, Donaldson LJ, Burn J. Limb reduction defects in the Northern Region of England 1985-1992.
37. Department of Health. *On the State of the Public Health: the annual report of the Chief Medical Officer of the Department of Health for the year 1993.* London: HMSO, 1994; 136.
38. Gene Therapy Advisory Committee. *Guidance on making proposals to conduct gene therapy research on human subjects.* London: Department of Health, 1994. Chair: Professor Dame June Lloyd.
39. Department for Education, Welsh Office. *Code of practice on the identification and assessment of special educational needs.* London: Central Office of Information, 1994.
40. *Education Act 1993.* London: HMSO, 1993.
41. Department for Education, Department of Health. *The education of children with emotional and behavioural difficulties.* London: Department for Education, Department of Health, 1994 (DFE Circular: 9/94, DH Local Authority Circular: LAC(94)9).
42. Department for Education, Department of Health. *The education of sick children.* London: Department for Education, Department of Health, 1994 (DFE Circular: 12/94, DH Local Authority Circular: LAC(94)10, Health Service Guidelines: HSG(94)24).
43. Department for Education, Department of Health. *The education of children being looked after by Local Authorities.* London: Department for Education, Department of Health, 1994 (DFE Circular: 13/94, DH Local Authority Circular: LAC(94)11).

(i)   Learning disabilities

The objectives of the Health of the Nation strategy[1] are relevant to people with learning disabilities, and a booklet which looks at ways to ensure that people with learning disabilities are included in action taken for the whole population has been prepared for publication early in 1995. It looks at services to support people with learning disabilities which are needed to achieve the aims of the policy. The booklet also mentions the health of carers.

The Advisory Group on services for people with learning disabilities and challenging behaviour or mental health needs undertook a programme of work to develop the ability of purchasers (local authority social services departments, DHAs, and GP fundholders) to commission services for this client group. A series of regional workshops was followed by topic-based working groups, which will report to a national conference early in 1995.

In October, the Standing Medical Advisory Committee revised its advice about atlanto-axial instability in people with Down's syndrome, in the light of new evidence about the unreliability of radiological examination for this condition.

An Advisory Group was established to support the work of the Chief Nursing Officer's initiative on learning disability nursing.

Reference

1. Department of Health. *The Health of the Nation: a strategy for health in England.* London: HMSO, 1992 (Cm. 1986).

154

(j)   Disability and rehabilitation

During 1994, there were further developments in the areas of disability and rehabilitation. National Continence Week was held in March to increase awareness of and to help remove some of the taboos that surround this subject. A further Continence Day will be held on 21 March 1995.

In June, the NHS Executive set out priorities for the NHS in 1995/96[1]. Local purchasers of services were asked to improve services for people with physical disabilities.

In July, following last year's publication of *Pressure sores: a key quality indicator*[2], the Department issued a leaflet[3] for patients and informal carers to advise about how to prevent pressure sores. Later in the year, work began on producing a video on pressure sore prevention for care assistants in residential care and nursing homes.

DH continued to fund 12 projects to improve NHS rehabilitation services for people who have suffered brain injury. A conference was arranged at which representatives of the projects reviewed progress; a report of this conference was circulated to the NHS and social services departments[4].

Research projects on the development of measurable targets were established in six areas: improvement of services to people with speech and language impairment; pressure sores; quality of care of hip fracture patients; avoidable amputations in diabetic patients; hearing disability; and urinary incontinence.

There was close consultation with the NHS about the devolution to the NHS of the DH budget for the supply of environmental control systems which assist people with severe disability to control their environment.
.
The Advisory Group on rehabilitation met on four occasions.

References

1.   Department of Health. *Priorities and planning guidance for the NHS: 1995/96.* Heywood (Lancashire): Department of Health, 1994 (Executive Letter: EL(94)55).
2.   Department of Health. *Pressure sores: a key quality indicator: a guide for NHS purchasers and providers.* Heywood (Lancashire): Department of Health, 1993.
3.   Department of Health. *Relieving the pressure: your guide to pressure sores.* Heywood (Lancashire): Department of Health, 1994.
4.   Department of Health. *Report of the brain injury rehabilitation conference, Peterborough, March 1994.* Heywood (Lancashire): Department of Health, 1994.

(k)   Prison health care

As in previous years, the Directorate of Health Care for Prisoners has operated within the context of continued change in the Prison Service and in the NHS, on which prisons increasingly depend for services. One of the most radical and important changes has been the devolution of responsibility for the effective delivery of health care to prisoners from the Directorate to prison managers at local level; the Directorate retains its policy role and has also taken on responsibility for health and safety within the Prison Service. This entails not only the statutory regulations for fire safety and health and safety at work, but also the occupational health of staff.

Reflecting these changes, the Directorate has made substantive changes in personnel and structure and has established a vision for the future "... of safe and healthy settings for prisoners, staff and visitors; with health care services which meet the needs of prisoners and staff and achieve a standard of excellence acknowledged throughout the world"[1].

Priorities during 1994 have included the introduction of strategic planning as a core function both locally and centrally, with greater contracting in of health service provision. Two further Health Care Standards have been published, to add to the previous six.

In the Spring, the Prison Service drugs strategy was launched - a strategic priority for the Prison Service, and in the forefront of the Government's national drugs strategy. The Prison Service drugs strategy focuses on three elements: control of the supply of illegal drugs in prisons; reduction in demand for drugs of abuse; and reduction of drug-associated health risks. The Directorate's provision of addiction treatment programmes should ensure that all inmates will have access to suitable treatment.

Other initiatives include policy development towards designation as a World Health Organization (WHO) collaborating centre for health promoting prisons, a review of medical staffing and the design of an enhanced health information database.

A key aspect of future health care in the Prison Service is collaboration with professional bodies in the development of training for doctors, nurses and other health care staff. Education and career development are recognised as vital components in the recruitment and retention of staff of high calibre.

Areas of joint work with DH and the NHS include increased collaboration in pilot contracts for mental health, and for genito-urinary medicine (GUM) services, the primary care contract, communicable diseases surveillance and local reviews of health care services, which included one at HMP Holloway.

Reference

1.   Directorate of Health Care for Prisoners. *Health care standards for prisons in England and Wales.* London: HM Prison Service, 1994.

(l)   London Implementation Group

The London Implementation Group (LIG) continued to encourage improvements in primary and community care services within the London Initiative Zone (LIZ). Between the financial years 1993/94 and 1994/95, an extra £125 million were invested in the LIZ, in addition to resources allocated to primary care by local health agencies. As a result, nearly 1,000 schemes are planned or under way in the LIZ to improve family doctor and community health services and premises.

Initial development plans identified the need to raise the basic standards of premises and the availability of staff for primary care in inner London as a key priority. In 1994/95, there has been greater emphasis on the shift from hospital to community care, to make better use of hospital beds and to promote new ways of working. Some £20 million were specifically targeted on projects to achieve this objective; one-quarter of this sum was used to improve services for the mentally ill.

In 1993/94, £7.5 million was set aside to fund, over three years, the contribution made by voluntary sector schemes which facilitate early discharge and help to avoid inappropriate admissions to hospital. The London Health Partnership, an alliance of charitable foundations, business interests and Government, was launched in June, to promote the development of urban primary care over the next three to five years.

The Primary Care Support Force for London was set up in October to help those involved in the local day-to-day management and delivery of services within the LIZ to advance the primary care development programme. It will also help to identify innovative ways of working and to ensure that such good practice is shared with others. The Secretary of State for Health announced that, from 1 April, there would be 13 further NHS Trusts in greater London. A number of NHS Trusts continued to develop plans for the concentration of hospital services onto fewer sites.

East London and the City Health Authority began public consultation in November on proposals to concentrate the services provided by the Royal Hospitals Trust (which includes St Bartholomew's Hospital and the London Chest Hospital) at the Royal London Hospital, Whitechapel; to develop the Homerton Hospital as a full district general hospital; and to close Queen Elizabeth Hospital, Hackney, and transfer its services to multi-specialty sites at the Homerton and Royal London Hospitals.

Lambeth, Southwark and Lewisham Health Commission began public consultation in November on proposals to consolidate inpatient and specialist services at St Thomas's Hospital; to use Guy's Hospital as an ambulatory care centre - including day surgery, treatment of minor injuries, outpatients departments and elective surgery; to provide an additional 60 beds at King's College Hospital to improve the handling of emergency admissions and to develop, in conjunction with the Maudsley Hospital, a specialist neurosciences centre; and to develop the Queen Elizabeth Military Hospital as the main acute hospital for Greenwich, with Regional specialties currently provided at the Brook Hospital to transfer to the King's Healthcare Trust (neurosciences and some cardiac surgery) and the Guy's and St Thomas' Hospital Trust (most cardiac surgery).

Substantial investments have recently been made or agreed to develop acute services at major hospitals in London, including a £28.3 million redevelopment of Lewisham Hospital to provide better facilities for children, maternity services, accident and emergency and elderly patients; a £19 million development at the Homerton Hospital, Hackney, to expand accident and emergency services and create a new facility for mentally ill people; a £2 million scheme at the Whittington Hospital to expand accident and emergency and associated services; a £6.5 million scheme to relocate St Mark's Hospital into refurbished accommodation at Northwick Park Hospital; and an £8.2 million scheme to expand and upgrade accident and emergency facilities at King's College Hospital.

Progress has been made with the medical school mergers recommended in the Tomlinson Report[1]. Firm agreement in principle to merger has been made by all of the undergraduate medical schools concerned, the Royal Postgraduate Medical School, and by five of the seven constituent institutes of the British Postgraduate Medical Federation. The Higher Education Funding Council for England has decided to set aside £80 million between the financial years 1995/96 and 1997/98 for projects to implement *Making London better*[2].

References

1. Department of Health, Department for Education. *Report of the Inquiry into London's Health Service, Medical Education and Research: presented to the Secretary of State for Health and Education by Sir Bernard Tomlinson.* London: HMSO, 1992.
2. Department of Health. *Making London better.* Heywood (Lancashire): Department of Health, 1993.

CHAPTER 6

COMMUNICABLE DISEASES

(a)   HIV infection and AIDS

Government strategy on HIV infection and AIDS

The main aims of the Government's strategy on HIV infection and AIDS are to limit the further spread of HIV infection, and to ensure that resources and services are properly targeted, that the right balance is struck with other health priorities, and that initiatives to combat HIV infection and AIDS are brought within the mainstream of health care and health promotion.

Progress of the epidemic

AIDS

Surveillance of the epidemic is implemented through the voluntary confidential reporting systems operated by the Public Health Laboratory Service (PHLS) AIDS Centre at the Communicable Disease Surveillance Centre (CDSC)[1,2] and the Government's programme of unlinked anonymous HIV surveys, implemented by the PHLS AIDS Centre[3].

Details of the number of AIDS cases reported in England are shown in Table 6.1 and Figure 6.1. 1,634 cases of AIDS were reported in England in 1994: these brought the cumulative total of AIDS cases reported since 1982 to 9,510, of whom 6,434 are known to have died. It is estimated that, on average, people newly diagnosed with AIDS were infected with HIV 10 years previously. Figure 6.2 compares the United Kingdom (UK) cumulative rate per million population to September 1994 with other Member States in the European Community (EC).

HIV infection

Table 6.2 and Figure 6.3 show details of reports of the 2,204 people with newly diagnosed HIV infection in England, bringing the cumulative total of such reports since 1984 to 20,440. Many factors might influence the decision to be tested for HIV infection, and these reports provide an incomplete indication of the true cumulative number of HIV infections. Evidence of new HIV infection and continued high-risk behaviour among homosexual men is of particular concern[3]: men who have sex with men continue to predominate among reports of HIV infections and AIDS.

Unlinked anonymous surveillance

Unlinked anonymous surveys were set up in January 1990 to supplement data available from voluntary confidential testing and to permit a more accurate

Table 6.1: *AIDS cases and known deaths by exposure category and date of report, England, 1982-31 December 1994*
(Numbers subject to revision as further data are received or duplicates identified)

How persons probably acquired the virus	Jan 1993-Dec 1993 Cases		Jan 1994-Dec 1994 Cases		Jan 1982-Dec 1994 Male		Female	
	Male	Female	Male	Female	Cases	Deaths	Cases	Deaths
Sexual intercourse:								
Between men	1007	-	1092	-	7095	4970	-	-
Between men and women								
'High risk' partner*	4	21	6	16	31	16	82	48
Other partner abroad**	108	94	137	97	553	301	378	180
Other partner UK	17	10	12	9	54	32	41	28
Partner risk not known	2	-	11	3	15	4	3	-
Injecting drug use (IDU)	44	29	68	24	255	154	111	59
IDU and sexual intercourse								
Between men	22	-	26	-	154	97	-	-
Blood								
Blood factor (eg haemophiliacs)	49	-	65	-	407	341	5	3
Blood or tissue transfer (eg transfusion)								
Abroad	3	12	2	2	12	5	40	23
UK	3	2	2	3	19	14	21	18
Mother to child	11	12	22	22	67	35	68	32
Other/undetermined	11	2	10	5	83	64	16	10
Total	1281	182	1453	181	8745	6033	765	401

* Men and women who had sex with injecting drug users, or with those infected through blood factor treatment or blood transfusion, and women who had sex with bisexual men.
** Includes persons without other identified risks who are from, or who have lived in, countries where the major route of HIV-1 transmission is through sexual intercourse between men and women.

Source: CDSC

Figure 6.1: *AIDS cases: total numbers and numbers where infection was probably acquired through sexual intercourse between men and women, England, to 31 December 1994*

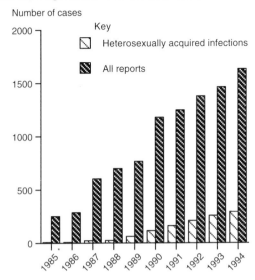

Number of cases

Key
- ⬜ Heterosexually acquired infections
- ⬛ All reports

* 1985 or earlier

Source: CDSC

Figure 6.2: *Reported AIDS cases in Europe: cumulative rates per million population to September 1994*

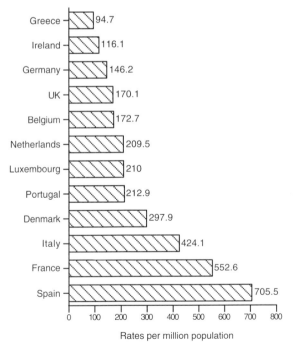

Greece — 94.7
Ireland — 116.1
Germany — 146.2
UK — 170.1
Belgium — 172.7
Netherlands — 209.5
Luxembourg — 210
Portugal — 212.9
Denmark — 297.9
Italy — 424.1
France — 552.6
Spain — 705.5

Rates per million population

Source: European Centre for the Epidemiological Monitoring of AIDS

Table 6.2: HIV antibody-positive people by exposure category and date of report, England, to 31 December 1994
(Numbers subject to revision as further data are received or duplicates identified)

How persons probably acquired the virus	Jan 1993-Dec 1993			Jan 1994-Dec 1994			Nov 1984-Dec 1994		
	Male	Female	NK†	Male	Female	NK†	Male	Female	NK†
Sexual intercourse:									
Between men	1293	-	-	1250	-	-	13063	-	-
Between men and women									
'High risk' partner*	6	56	-	9	27	-	66	323	-
Other partner abroad**	240	231	-	230	254	1	1369	1290	5
Other partner UK	23	25	-	23	29	-	95	162	-
Partner risk not known	6	5	1	18	25	-	43	46	-
Injecting drug use (IDU)	103	38	-	106	49	-	1093	500	3
IDU and sexual intercourse between men	23	-	-	26	-	-	292	-	-
Blood									
Blood factor (eg haemophiliacs)	3	-	-	4	-	-	1062	10	-
Blood or tissue transfer (eg transfusion)									
Abroad/UK	3	3	-	5	8	-	59	67	1
Mother to child‡	25	38	-	22	19	1	128	124	1
Other/undetermined	47	9	2	80	18	-	523	84	31
Total	1772	405	3	1773	429	2	17793	2606	41

† NK = Not known (sex not stated on report).

* Men and women who had sex with injecting drug users, or with those infected through blood factor treatment or blood transfusion, and women who had sex with bisexual men.

**Includes persons without other identified risks who are from, or who have lived in, countries where the major route of HIV-1 transmission is through sexual intercourse between men and women.

‡ By date of report that established infected status of infant.

Source: CDSC

162

Figure 6.3: *HIV antibody-positive people: total numbers and numbers where infection was probably acquired through sexual intercourse between men and women, England, by year of report to 31 December 1994*

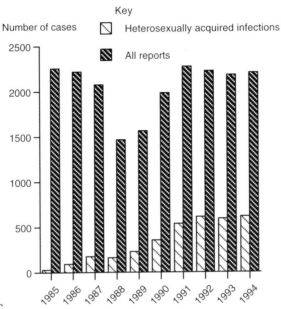

Source: CDSC

picture of the epidemic. The surveys are established in a number of genito-urinary medicine (GUM) clinics, centres for injecting drug misusers and antenatal clinics; screening of dried blood spots from neonates also takes place. Publication of a report from the Unlinked Anonymous HIV Surveys Steering Group with results to end-1993 is expected in early 1995.

Preliminary results are summarised in Table 6.3 and show that, whilst prevalence is highest in London, HIV-1 infection is present in high-risk groups in every region surveyed. Prevalence rates in 1993 among homosexual or bisexual men attending GUM clinics were 16% in London and the South-East compared with 4% elsewhere. Of particular concern is the high prevalence in those under 25 years-of-age, which indicates continuing transmission.

Prevalence rates among injecting drug misusers were 4.0% for men and 2.8% for women in London and the South-East, and less than 1% in men and women elsewhere. This group remain vulnerable because younger users report the sharing of drug-injecting equipment.

In London there was a striking rise in HIV-1 prevalence among pregnant women between 1990 and 1993 (see Figure 6.4), from 1 in 1,220 in 1990 to 1 in 570 in 1993. Data from other sources indicate that the higher prevalence in London may be linked to exposure to infection in Africa. Comparison of data from these surveys with reported births to HIV-1-infected mothers show that only 12% of infections have been clinically recognised.

Table 6.3: Prevalence of HIV-1 infection in unlinked anonymous survey groups, England and Wales, 1993

Survey group	London and South-East England*				England and Wales outside the South-East				Prevalence ratio‡ London vs elsewhere
	Number tested	Number HIV-1 infected	% HIV-1 infected	Prevalence range (%)†	Number tested	Number HIV-1 infected	% HIV-1 infected	Prevalence range (%)†	
Males									
Genito-urinary medicine clinic attenders:									
Homo/bisexual§	2691	425	15.79	3.61, 21.36	1601	69	4.31	0.73, 8.24	3.7
Heterosexual§	7197	70	0.97	0.08, 1.86	18019	20	0.11	0, 0.30	8.8
Injecting drug users attending agencies#	571	23	4.0	0.90, 8.80	1909	11	0.58	0, 1.50	6.9
Females									
Genito-urinary medicine clinic attenders:									
Heterosexual§	9870	56	0.57	0.28, 1.16	15834	14	0.09	0, 0.49	6.3
Injecting drug users attending agencies#	217	6	2.76	2.40, 3.20	674	5	0.74	0.40, 2.90	3.7
Pregnant women at delivery (infant dried blood spots)**	103092	182	0.18	0, 0.52	140735	6	0.004	0, 0.06	41.4
Pregnant women seeking terminations	8209	40	0.49	0.21, 0.88	-	-	-	-	-

* The injecting drug user survey includes data from a few agencies in the South-East outside London; all other surveys present data for London.

† The range within a category is the lowest and highest rates recorded in individual clinics (GUM survey), regions (injecting drug users survey), districts (infant dried blood spot survey) or hospitals (termination of pregnancy and antenatal surveys).

§ Excluding known drug users.

Attending specialist centres for injecting drug users.

** Prevalence in South-East England outside London was 0.02% in 1993. In Northern and Yorkshire Region data for pregnant women come from the antenatal survey.

‡ The ratio by which the prevalence of infection in London is greater than the prevalence in England and Wales outside the South-East.

Source: Unlinked Anonymous HIV Surveys

Figure 6.4: *Trends in prevalence of HIV-1 infection among pregnant women by area of residence, England, 1988-93*

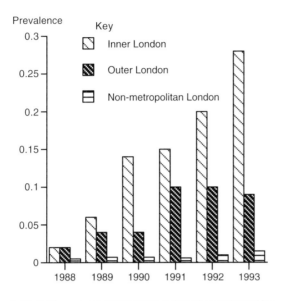

Source: Survey in North Thames and South Thames (West) co-ordinated by
Institute of Child Health, London; survey in South Thames (East)
co-ordinated by PHLS AIDS Centre (commenced in 1992)

Table 6.4: *HIV in blood donations in the United Kingdom, October 1985 to December 1994*

Year	Donations tested (million)	Donations confirmed HIV-seropositive			
		Male	Female	Total	%
1985	0.6	13	0	13	0.002
1986	2.64	44	9	53	0.002
1987	2.59	18	5	23	0.0009
1988	2.64	18	5	23	0.0009
1989	2.74	25	12	37	0.001
1990	2.82	23*	12	35*	0.001
1991	2.95	23	8	31	0.001
1992	2.90	15	11	26	0.0009
1993	2.92	16	4	20	0.0007
1994	2.91	8	8	16	0.0005
Total	*25.71*	*203*	*74*	*277*	*0.001*

*Includes one anti-HIV-2-positive donation.

Source: National Blood Authority

AIDS/HIV infected health care workers

In March, DH published revised guidance[4] on the management of HIV-infected health care workers, based on the recommendations of the Expert Advisory Group on AIDS. This guidance incorporates new ethics statements from professional regulatory bodies.

A Working Group met during 1994 to review the risk of HIV transmission from health care workers to patients, informed by an independent review of published research. The Group will report to the UK Advisory Panel for health care workers infected with bloodborne viruses in 1995.

HIV in blood donations

During 1994, 2.91 million blood donations in the UK were tested with anti-HIV-1+2 combined tests. Sixteen donations (from 8 males and 8 females) were found to be HIV-seropositive, a rate of 1 in 182,106 (0.0005%). The number of new donors tested was 352,000, of whom 10 were seropositive (1 in 35,200 [0.003%]). Again, no donations were found to be anti-HIV-2 positive during 1994.

Table 6.4 shows the number of donations tested in the UK between the Autumn of 1985 and the end of 1994, together with the number of donations confirmed as HIV-seropositive. The male:female ratio of seropositive donations in 1994 was 1 to 1, as it was for new donors. This is the first year in which there have been as many female seropositive donors as male.

Guidelines for offering voluntary named HIV antibody testing to women receiving antenatal care

Revised guidance was published in June[5] to clarify and amplify advice given in an earlier document[6]. It reiterates the Department's policy to offer and to encourage HIV testing among all women attending for antenatal care in areas of high HIV prevalence, and includes updated HIV prevalence figures for pregnant women. The importance of staff training is emphasised.

Public education and prevention

The Health of the Nation White Paper[7] reaffirmed the need for concerted action nationally and locally, involving both statutory and voluntary agencies. The Government reviewed its overall HIV/AIDS policy and strategy in June 1993 to ensure that resources are properly targeted, and that HIV and AIDS policies operate within the mainstream of health promotion and health care services.

The Health Education Authority (HEA) has continued to produce materials to clarify information about HIV transmission and other sexually transmitted diseases (STDs), use of condoms and the negotiation of safer sex. The HEA also has targeted campaigns for ethnic minorities and for men who have sex with men or with men and women.

The National AIDS Helpline (NAH) has played a valuable role from the outset of the Government's HIV strategy. Following a review in 1993, a new service, which begins on 1 April 1995, will integrate operation of the NAH with a new National Drug Helpline, although the services will remain distinct.

Following a multi-faith consultation day held in July 1993, a national conference took place in March 1994. A resource book of information which has come to light because of the initiative will be produced by Summer 1995.

Paris AIDS Summit

In December, 42 countries signed the Paris AIDS Summit declaration. Ministers announced that an extra £2 million of Overseas Development Administration (ODA) funds would be committed to HIV/AIDS research over the next 3 years. Research will be supported on vaccine and microbicide development, in collaboration with the Medical Research Council (MRC), and on improving strategies for HIV prevention and cost-effective care.

References

1. Public Health Laboratory Service AIDS Centre. The surveillance of HIV-1 infection and AIDS in England and Wales. *Commun Dis Rep* 1991; **1**: R51-R56.
2. Wight PA, Rush AM, Miller E. Surveillance of HIV infection by voluntary testing in England. *Commun Dis Rep CDR Rev* 1992; **2**: R85-R90.
3. Evans BG, Catchpole MA, Heptonstall J et al., Sexually transmitted diseases and HIV-1 infection among homosexual men in England and Wales. *BMJ* 1993; **306**: 426-8.
4. UK Health Departments. *AIDS-HIV infected health care workers: guidance on the management of infected health care workers*. Heywood (Lancashire): Department of Health, 1994 (Health Service Guidelines: HSG (94)16).
5. Department of Health. *Guidelines for offering voluntary named HIV antibody testing to women receiving antenatal care*. Heywood (Lancashire): Department of Health, 1994 (Professional Letter: PL/CO(94)3).
6. Department of Health. *Guidelines for offering voluntary named HIV antibody testing to women receiving antenatal care*. Heywood (Lancashire): Department of Health, 1994 (Professional Letter: PL/CO(92)5).
7. Department of Health. *The Health of the Nation: a strategy for health in England*. London: HMSO, 1992 (Cm. 1986).

(b)   Other sexually transmitted diseases

The total number of new cases seen in GUM clinics in England continued to rise, with 661,261 seen in 1993, an increase of 0.7% over 1992 (see Table 6.5); these figures represent a fall of 1.7% among men and a rise of 2.1% in women. STDs and other infections requiring treatment were diagnosed in 53.5% overall (in 50% of men and 57% of women). Numbers of patients for whom no treatment was required or referral elsewhere was indicated also continued to rise. Overall, the number of reports of confirmed STDs and other infections fell by 2.5% from 362,940 to 353,752. Of these, approximately 24% were for wart virus infection, 17% for non-specific genital infection, 9% for *Chlamydia*, 7% for herpes simplex virus, 3% for gonorrhoea and 1.7% for pelvic inflammatory disease (PID). All figures are derived from the KC60 reporting form for consultations in NHS GUM clinics; cases diagnosed and managed without reference to GUM clinics are therefore not included, and the comparisons below are with previous KC60 data.

Table 6.5: *Sexually transmitted diseases reported by NHS genito-urinary medicine clinics, England, in year ending 31 December 1993*

Condition	Males	Females	Persons
All syphilis	892	455	1347
Infectious syphilis	*229*	*108*	*337*
All gonorrhoea	7318	4485	11803
Post-pubertal uncomplicated	*6534*	*3377*	*9911*
All chlamydia (excluding PID and chlamydial infections with arthritis)[1]	15785	17482	33267
Post-pubertal uncomplicated chlamydia	*12168*	*14053*	*26221*
Pelvic infection and epididymitis	1314	6295	7609
Non-specific urethritis (NSU) and related disease	44231	15879	60110
Chlamydial infections/NSU with arthritis	241	33	274
Chancroid/Donovanosis/LGV	28	12	40
Trichomoniasis	301	4967	5268
Vaginosis/vaginitis/balanitis	10887	36654	47541
Candidiasis	8858	50044	58902
Scabies/pediculosis	3788	1156	4944
All Herpes simplex	11637	13865	25502
Herpes simplex-first attack	*6247*	*8374*	*14621*
Herpes simplex-recurrence	*5390*	*5491*	*10881*
All Wart virus infection	48972	35748	84720
Wart virus infection-first attack	*25859*	*23034*	*48893*
Wart virus infection-recurrence	*23113*	*12714*	*35827*
Viral hepatitis	558	124	682
Asymptomatic HIV infection - first presentation	1001	219	1220
Asymptomatic HIV infection - subsequent presentation	*8945*	*1109*	*10054*
HIV infection with symptoms, not AIDS - first presentation	1411	206	1617
AIDS - first presentation	1001	116	1117
Other conditions requiring treatment[2]	63177	57917	121094
Other episodes not requiring treatment	96389	84194	180583
Other conditions referred elsewhere	6616	7005	13621
Total number of new cases seen	324405	336856	661261

[1] Comprises 'uncomplicated chlamydial infection', 'other complicated chlamydia (excluding PID and epididymitis)' and 'Chlamydia ophthalmia neonatorum'.

[2] Includes epidemiological treatment of trichomoniasis, vaginosis, vaginitis, balanitis and candidiasis.

LGV = lymphogranuloma venereum; PID = pelvic inflammatory disease.

Source: Form KC60

Figure 6.5: *All gonorrhoea: number of new cases seen at NHS genito-urinary medicine clinics, England, 1980-93*

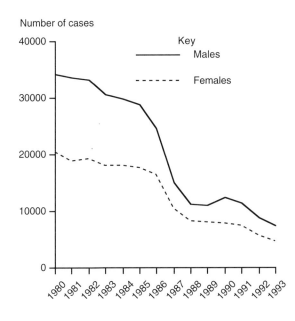

Source: Forms SBH60 and KC60

In 1993, total reports of gonorrhoea fell by 17% compared with 1992, from 14,283 to 11,803 (a decrease of 16% in men and 19% in women). A target set by the Health of the Nation strategy[1], to reduce the incidence of gonorrhoea among men and women aged 15-64 years by at least 20% by 1995 (ie, from 61 cases per 100,000 in 1990 to no more than 49 cases per 100,000) had already been achieved in 1992, when the rate in this age-group fell to 45 cases per 100,000 population; this rate was further reduced to 38 per 100,000 in 1993 (see Figure 6.5).

The total number of reports of uncomplicated chlamydial infection fell by 6.0% to 33,267, by 5.3% in men and 6.7% in women. Uncomplicated non-specific genital infections fell by 7.4% from 64,930 in 1992 to 60,110 in 1993; this figure includes an 8.5% fall in non-specific urethritis in men. There was a fall of 2.2% in reports of PID among women, from 6,437 in 1992 to 6,295 in 1993.

There was a slight increase in reports of syphilis (2.7%), entirely due to an increase of 8.7% for non-infectious syphilis in men; there was no change in reports of infectious syphilis (337 cases in 1993 compared with 338 in 1992).

First attacks of herpes simplex virus (HSV) infection rose by 1.7% in men to 6,247 cases and by 6.3% in women to 8,374 cases, an overall rise of 4.3%. First attacks of HSV are now more common in women, accounting for 57% of such

Table 6.6: Sexually transmitted diseases reported by NHS GUM clinics in England, 1993, by age (in years)

Condition	Sex	All ages	Under 16	16-19	20-24	25-34	35-44	45 and over	Estimated median age
Infectious syphilis	M	229	1	6	22	99	50	51	33
	F	108	0	14	22	41	24	7	29
Post-pubertal uncomplicated gonorrhoea	M	6534	18	847	1859	2900	684	226	26
	F	3377	90	1096	1082	915	152	42	22
Post-pubertal uncomplicated chlamydia	M	12168	25	1097	4313	5242	1139	352	26
	F	14053	237	4045	5518	3567	552	135	22
Herpes simplex - first attack	M	6247	11	448	1520	2803	942	523	29
	F	8374	81	1498	2711	2916	830	338	24
Wart virus infection - first attack	M	25859	81	2057	9464	10510	2538	1209	26
	F	23034	317	5826	8623	6073	1519	676	23

Source: Form KC60

reports. Reports of recurrent attacks of HSV rose by 12.7% in women, accounting for a 5.3% increase overall; recurrent attacks accounted for 43% of all reports of HSV infection during 1993.

There were falls in first attacks of viral warts among men (4.8%) and women (3.8%); however, total reports of viral warts remained roughly constant as there were increased reports of recurrent attacks of 3.7% in men and 13.6% in women. Recurrent attacks accounted for 42% of all reports of wart virus infection during 1993.

A high proportion of reports of STDs come from patients in younger age groups (see Table 6.6).

Reference

1. Department of Health. *The Health of the Nation: a strategy for health in England*. London: HMSO, 1992 (Cm. 1986).

(c)   Immunisation

Measles/rubella immunisation campaign

Epidemiology

After five years of excellent control of measles, it became clear in 1994 that measles notifications were rising and that the pattern of measles was changing. More cases were occurring in outbreaks and these were increasingly among older children (see Figure 6.6).

Laboratory confirmation of measles showed that the distribution of cases was indeed shifting to older groups. Figure 6.7 provides an estimate of the probability that notified cases were correctly diagnosed. When this probability was applied to the notified cases according to their age, it could be seen that the age-group at highest risk of measles was not that group from whom most notifications were coming (children aged under 9 years), but rather children aged 10-14 years (see Figure 6.8).

Guided by the above epidemiological findings, and by experience from Scotland, where a measles epidemic had already started in late 1993/early 1994, and taking account of the predictions from two independent groups using mathematical models that a large epidemic was likely by 1996/97, the Joint Committee on Vaccination and Immunisation (JCVI) recommended a nationwide school-based immunisation campaign. JCVI also recommended that the vaccine of choice was measles/rubella (MR) vaccine. The inclusion of rubella vaccine was recommended on the grounds of an already identified susceptibility in teenagers, especially males, among whom there had been a large number of rubella infections in 1993. The target population, all schoolchildren aged 5-16 years, was chosen on the basis of age-specific sero-epidemiology that identified this group as most likely to benefit from immunisation, and matched well the planned

Figure 6.6: *Measles notifications, England and Wales, 1988-94*

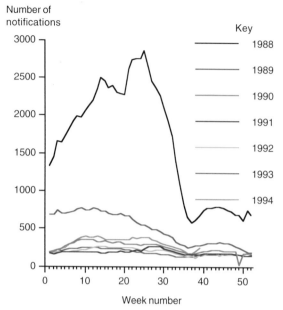

Source: OPCS

Figure 6.7: *Proportion of notified measles cases confirmed by laboratory testing, by age-group, England and Wales, 1993-94*

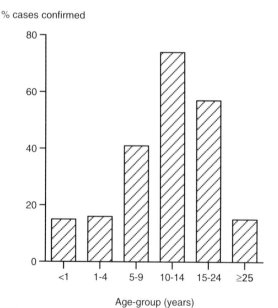

Source: PHLS

Figure 6.8: *Notifications of measles, and notifications 'corrected' by probability of correct diagnosis, by age-group, England and Wales, 1993-94*

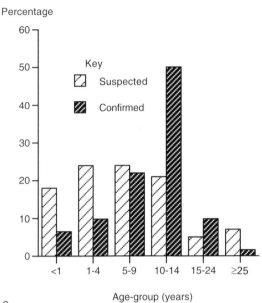

Source: PHLS

immunisation of schoolchildren. In view of rising reports of measles (see Figure 6.6) and the experience in Scotland, it was decided that the campaign needed to be implemented in November 1994, a year earlier than had previously been identified.

Implementation

In the Summer, an implementation group was set up under the chairmanship of Dr Stephen Horsley, Regional Director of Public Health of North Western RHA. In July, the NHS Executive Board agreed that the campaign should be implemented through the NHS in November; costs of vaccine, distribution and national publicity were borne by DH.

Postcodes of 27,000 schools were provided by the Department for Education (DFE). These were re-aggregated according to DHAs and issued to district immunisation co-ordinators. Co-ordinators obtained school rolls for each school and these formed the basis for identification of the target population: these figures were submitted to DH and used for allocation of vaccine.

Around 12 million doses of vaccine were issued in advance of the campaign, with every DHA appropriately resourced for vaccine and the means to give it by the start of the campaign. There were no supply problems. Most DHAs ran their campaigns during November, with mop-up activities in December. In some cases, the campaign ran through December with mop-up activities to be completed by early February.

Results

The target population for England was 7.17 million children. The first returns from DHAs and NHS Trusts reported on the number of children immunised during November alone, with a national uptake around 90%. Final returns for the November phase and the mop-up activities show immunisation of 92% of the target 7.1 million children aged 5-16 years (see Table 6.7).

Notifications in 1994 had been rising in line with those seen in 1987, shortly before the 1988 measles epidemic; in 1988, the last epidemic year, there were 86,000 notifications. The predictions for 1995 had suggested an epidemic of some 150,000 cases; because more of these infections would have occurred in older individuals than in the previous epidemic, and measles case-fatality rates increase with advancing age, approximately 50 deaths were anticipated. By contrast with these predictions, measles notifications following the immunisation campaign have fallen (see Figures 6.9 and 6.10).

Previous experience indicates that measles notification data may show useful trends but individual notifications are highly unreliable, especially in younger children; the specificity of notification among children aged under 5 years is well below 20%. Since the beginning of November 1994, however, the PHLS has been able to use salivary antibody testing to confirm measles in suspected cases. There were more than 100 positive reports in November and December 1994. Early data from 1995 indicate only 24 confirmed measles cases from 2,700 samples, mainly outside the age-groups targeted in the campaign (see Figure 6.11).

Suspected adverse reactions

Before the start of the campaign, the post-licensing division of the Medicines Control Agency (MCA) agreed that all suspected MR vaccine adverse reactions would be handled as the highest priority. Yellow card reports were classified and entered into the MCA database within 36 hours of receipt. The MCA

Table 6.7: *Immunisation coverage for the measles/rubella campaign, by District Health Authority/NHS Trust, England, 1994*

Coverage(%)	DHAs/Trusts (%)
>95	37 (21.5)
90-95	96 (55.8)
85-90	31 (18.0)
80-85	6 (3.5)
<80	2 (1.2)
Mean coverage: 92%	*Total: 172*

Source: DH

Figure 6.9: *Measles notifications as five-week moving averages, England and Wales, 1987 and 1994*

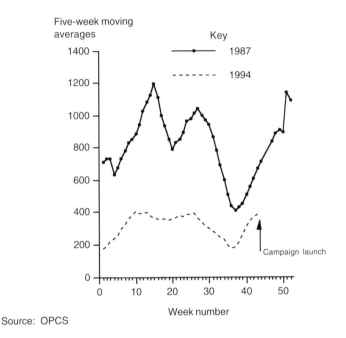

Source: OPCS

Figure 6.10: *Numbers of measles notifications, England and Wales, 1987-88 and 1994-95*

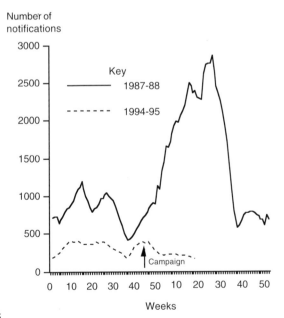

Source: OPCS

175

Figure 6.11: *Cases of measles confirmed by salivary antibody testing, England and Wales, 1994-95*

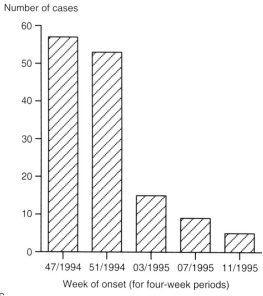

Source: PHLS

database was computer-linked with the measles team database and all reports relating to MR vaccine were transferred on a daily basis. Requests for more information have been sent to all doctors reporting serious adverse reactions.

Approximately 8 million children have been immunised in the UK campaign and the following results are for adverse reactions for the UK. The final figures for adverse reactions may differ slightly from those stated here because late-onset reactions are still being reported. 2,729 discrete adverse reactions have been reported in 1,187 children, an estimated rate of one affected child per 7,000 immunisations. Most of the reports were of minor conditions, many of which were unlikely to be linked to the immunisation, or of no likely consequence. 637 serious reactions were reported (more than one can occur in each child), but no deaths. Serious adverse reactions fell into two groups - those occurring immediately or soon after the immunisation, and those occurring later. There were 120 reports of immediate allergic-type reactions, such as anaphylaxis, bronchospasm or 'collapse'. Some children were admitted briefly to hospital, but no serious lasting effects or deaths were reported after these reactions. 114 significant 'neurological' reactions were reported, although some were probably unrelated to the immunisation. A number of convulsions occurred on the day of immunisation, and were thought to be either chance occurrences or precipitated by the emotion of the event. Three cases of Guillain-Barré syndrome were reported: one of these, a pure sensory form, is highly atypical. Other reports included erythema multiforme, Henoch-Schönlein purpura and arthritis/arthropathy. A more detailed analysis, including an estimate of causality, will be prepared when all the follow-up inquiries have been completed.

Evaluation

The impact of the campaign is being evaluated from coverage and surveillance data. The HEA has undertaken market research of the awareness and information gained from the advertisements: early reports suggest a very high awareness of the campaign publicity. Before the campaign, measles had been rated by the public as one of the least serious of all childhood infectious diseases. The main focus of the campaign was to highlight the potential seriousness of measles, and post-campaign evaluation suggests that parental awareness of the seriousness of measles had shifted considerably. Only 3% of the parents interviewed said that they had withheld consent; the commonest reason was that their child had already had measles or measles, mumps, and rubella (MMR) vaccines. This figure matches the DHA returns on refusal-to-consent rates.

In association with the Royal College of Nursing, a distance-learning module was prepared on the MR campaign, transmitted by BBC Select television and made available on video to all district co-ordinators. This and other information provided to nurses, and their impressions of the organisation of the campaign, are being evaluated by the Queen's Nursing Institute. The arrangements for supply of vaccine and consumables are also being audited.

Conclusion

In view of the short period of time available between the decision to run the campaign and its implementation, an enormous amount of preparation was necessary against very tight deadlines. There were some unexpected difficulties, such as the concern of some sections of the community about the origins of the cell-line used to grow rubella vaccine viruses; notwithstanding such problems, very high coverage was achieved within the allotted period.

The impact of the campaign is already apparent. A measles epidemic in 1995 now looks extremely unlikely and there are very real prospects that measles transmission will be interrupted in much of the country. JCVI will shortly be making recommendations on the next steps to consolidate the gains achieved.

A very large number of health professionals played their part in the campaign. General practitioners (GPs) clearly dealt with many inquiries from parents - a gratifying sign of the trust that parents have in their GPs as sources of such advice. Immunisation co-ordinators, school health services, pharmacists and many others also made invaluable contributions.

Other immunisations

Immunisation coverage has remained at satisfactory levels; the national target of 95% coverage was achieved for diphtheria, tetanus and polio vaccines in children reaching their second birthday. *Haemophilus influenzae* type b (Hib) vaccine coverage is 93%, and that for pertussis and MMR vaccines is 92%. Following

Figure 6.12: *Notifications of Haemophilus influenzae meningitis, England and Wales, 1989-95*

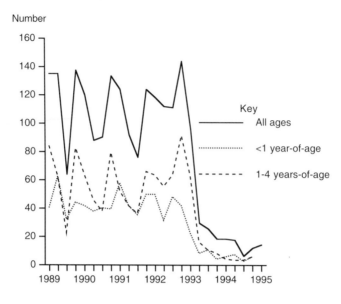

Source: OPCS

Figure 6.13: *Notifications of pertussis infection, England and Wales, 1940-94, and vaccination coverage, 1969-94*

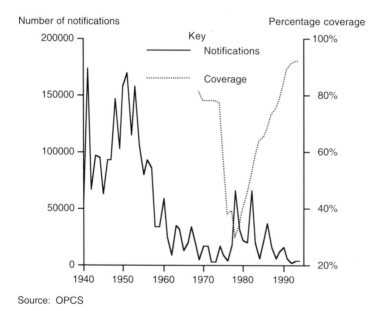

Source: OPCS

the introduction of Hib immunisation in 1992, notifications of *Haemophilus influenzae* meningitis continued to fall to very low levels (see Figure 6.12).

The cyclical pattern of four-yearly upsurges of pertussis appears to have been suppressed by the present high levels of immunisation (see Figure 6.13).

Despite the increasing numbers of reports of diphtheria from the former Soviet Union, there has been no significant evidence of importations into this country. In 1994, there were no reports of imported or vaccine-associated poliomyelitis; it is more than a decade since there were any reported cases caused by wild polio viruses.

(d)   Viral hepatitis

Viral hepatitis is a notifiable disease. In 1994 a provisional total of 3,734 cases were notified to the OPCS from England, a fall of 33% compared with the previous year. Of these 2,726 were due to hepatitis A and 532 due to hepatitis B. A further source of data is obtained through the voluntary confidential reporting by laboratories of confirmed cases to PHLS CDSC; provisional figures from this voluntary reporting system are discussed below.

Hepatitis A

The incidence of hepatitis A fluctuates. The most recent peak year for hepatitis A was 1990 when 7,248 cases were reported to CDSC from England. Reports have decreased in each of the past four years (see Figure 6.14), with 2,231 reports being received in 1994.

Most cases of hepatitis A infection seen in England are acquired in the UK and while most of these are sporadic, outbreaks do occur.

Travellers to countries with a high prevalence of hepatitis A may be at increased risk of contracting the virus. A history of travel abroad in the six weeks before the onset of the illness was recorded in 281 cases (13%) of cases reported to CDSC in 1994 (see page 189).

Hepatitis B

Much acute hepatitis B infection is subclinical, may not be diagnosed and therefore cannot be reported. The number of new hepatitis B infections in the UK is low.

CDSC received reports of 595 cases of acute hepatitis B diagnosed in England in 1994. Information about risk exposure was available in 353 (60%), among whom transmission was likely to have occurred as a result of sexual intercourse between men in 103, sexual intercourse between men and women in 96, injecting drug misuse in 96, and as a result of medical treatment or blood transfusion abroad in nine. Cases were also reported in infants born to hepatitis-B-surface-

Figure 6.14: *Reports of hepatitis A to CDSC, England, 1980-94*

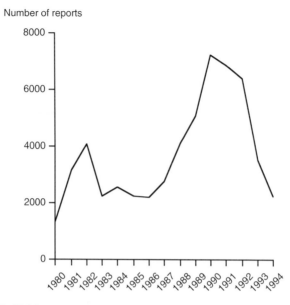

Number of reports

Source: PHLS, CDSC

Figure 6.15: *Reports of hepatitis B to CDSC (all reports and reports in injecting drug users), England, 1980-94*

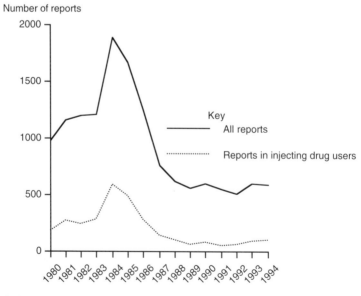

Number of reports

Key

All reports

Reports in injecting drug users

Source: PHLS, CDSC

Table 6.8: *Laboratory reports of acute hepatitis B virus infections in selected risk groups, England, 1985-94*

Risk group	1985	1986	1987	1988	1989	1990	1991	1992	1993	1994
Total	1669	1255	762	617	559	599	553	512	603	595
IDUs	486	280	144	102	65	80	55	59	95	96
Sex between men	123	105	54	49	38	82	88	95	87	103
IDUs/sex between men	10	4	-	2	2	3	1	1	-	-
Sex between men and women	149	140	79	67	44	77	68	80	56	96
Other	100	84	92	69	45	69	52	53	87	58
RNI	801	642	393	328	365	288	289	224	278	242

IDUs = intravenous drug users; RNI = risk not identified.

Source: PHLS, CDSC

antigen (HBsAg) positive mothers and who had not received complete courses of hepatitis B vaccine after birth.

Reports of acute hepatitis B peaked in 1984 and subsequently fell (see Figure 6.15); this decline occurred in most risk groups (see Table 6.8). In some, this may be linked to the modification of risk behaviours in response to the HIV/AIDS epidemic but in others, such as health care workers, the decrease probably reflects successful immunisation policy.

(e) Influenza

During the 1993-94 influenza season, influenza $A(H_3N_2)$, $A(H_1N_1)$ and influenza B all circulated world wide. However, $A(H_3N_2)$ viruses predominated; as many were antigenically distinct from the H_3N_2 strain in the 1993 vaccine, the World Health Organization (WHO) recommended a change in this component of the vaccine for the 1994-95 season.

At the beginning of December 1994, GP consultation rates for acute respiratory infections increased sharply and by the end of the year were the highest recorded since 1989. This increase was largely attributable to an increase in acute bronchitis (which includes acute bronchiolitis), especially among children aged 0-4 years. There was a concomitant increase in respiratory syncytial virus isolates. By the end of the year, laboratory reports of *Mycoplasma pneumoniae* infections had also increased. As in previous epidemics of this infection, which occur about every four years, the reports were mainly of infections in young adults and children.

GP consultations for influenza and influenza-like illness remained at low levels and although they were increasing slightly by the end of December they were still, at under 50 per 100,000 population, well within expected levels for the time of year. A few isolates of influenza B and an H_3N_2 subtype of influenza A, all covered by the vaccine, were confirmed by the Virus Reference Division at PHLS.

Several large studies from the United States of America published during the year supported the benefit of influenza immunisation in certain risk groups[1,2]. In the UK, up to 40-50% of those who are recommended for influenza vaccine each year currently receive it. In an attempt to improve uptake, GPs were encouraged in an early reminder in June's *CMO's Update*[3] to identify their at-risk patients and order vaccine for them well in advance. This would also allow more accurate determination of vaccine needs for the season. Just over 6 million doses of influenza vaccine were distributed - an 8% increase over 1993 - and no shortages or delays occurred.

References

1. Mulloolly JP. Influenza vaccination programmes for elderly persons: cost-effectiveness in a health maintenance organisation. *Ann Intern Med* 1994; **121**: 947-52.
2. Nichol KL. The efficacy and cost-effectiveness of vaccination against influenza among elderly persons living in the community. *N Engl J Med* 1994; **331**: 778-84.
3. Department of Health. Influenza immunisation. *CMO's Update* 1994; **3**: 1-2.

(f) Tuberculosis

A total of 5,694 cases of tuberculosis were provisionally notified in England and Wales in 1994, compared with 5,920 in 1993 and 5,798 in 1992. A more detailed analysis of routine notification data up to the end of 1993[1], together with preliminary data from the 1993 National Survey of Notifications of Tuberculosis in England and Wales[2], gave a clearer picture of recent trends. Between 1988 and 1993, total notifications for tuberculosis increased by 17%, such that by the end of 1993 an estimated 8,000 (95% confidence interval 2,988-11,967) more cases had been notified than would have been expected if the decline seen up to 1987 had continued. The increase was much more marked for non-respiratory (nearly 50% higher) than for respiratory (8.5% higher) disease.

Total tuberculosis notifications in the white population have fallen since 1988, with a fall in the annual notification rate in this group from 6.9 per 100,000 population in 1988 to 4.7 per 100,000 in 1993. In people originating from the Indian subcontinent, although total notifications rose, the notification rate continued to fall - from 175 per 100,000 in 1983 and 140 per 100,000 in 1988 to 128 per 100,000 in 1993. Notification rates also fell in people of West Indian origin, from 29 per 100,000 in 1988 to 20 per 100,000 in 1993. The most striking new trend revealed by the 1993 notification survey was a rise in the number of notifications in people of 'other' ethnic origin, particularly those of black African origin in whom the notification rate increased from 60.4 per 100,000 in 1988 to 128.9 per 100,000 in 1993.

The 1993 notification survey included an assessment of HIV prevalence in patients with tuberculosis aged 16 to 54 years by voluntary unlinked anonymous HIV testing. 40% of eligible patients were tested; of these, 2% were HIV positive. This is likely to be an underestimate, but does indicate that HIV infection is not at present a major contributing factor to tuberculosis in the UK.

Preliminary results of screening for tuberculosis at temporary Christmas shelters for the homeless in London in 1992 and 1993 showed that, among those who accepted on-site screening, tuberculosis was confirmed in 1.5% and suspected in a further 3.5% who were lost to follow-up (Kumar D, unpublished data). Homeless people are an important risk-group for tuberculosis, and their poor compliance with treatment is likely to prolong the period in which they can transmit the infection and to encourage the emergence of drug resistance. The screening campaign has since been extended to other homeless groups.

References

1   Hayward AC, Watson JM. Tuberculosis in England and Wales 1982-1993: notifications exceeded predictions. *Commun Dis Rep Review* (in press).
2.   Tuberculosis in 1993: preliminary results of national survey. *Commun Dis Rep Weekly* 1994; **4**: 235.

(g)   Plague

During September, reports were received of two outbreaks of plague in India. Although the public health threat to the UK was deemed to be small, DH mounted an immediate response, steered by a Task Force convened by the

Secretary of State for Health and the Chief Medical Officer. Liaison was co-ordinated across Government Departments and Agencies.

The Chief Medical Officer alerted all doctors so that they were aware of the symptoms of plague and to ensure that suspected cases and their contacts received prompt and appropriate investigation and treatment. Most doctors received the information within 48 hours via the new Public Health LINK electronic communication cascade for urgent messages[1]. Information was also disseminated rapidly to consultants in communicable disease control, infectious diseases units, and public health laboratories via the PHLS 'Epinet' system, and a surveillance protocol for suspected cases was established.

Controls at ports of entry were strengthened: information leaflets were provided to airlines and airports for issue to passengers and port health teams boarded aircraft from India to spray cabins and baggage to kill fleas. Port Health Authorities were advised on rodent and insect elimination and disinfection of ships, and importers were provided with advice on handling cargo. A comprehensive reference laboratory facility was set up via the PHLS Laboratory of Enteric Pathogens. No case of plague was identified in the UK.

Reference

1. Public Health LINK. *CMO's Update* 1994; **4:** 7.

(h)   Necrotising fasciitis

Between February and May, in Gloucestershire, seven people developed disease characteristic of invasive streptococcal infection, three of whom died. Five had confirmed and one had probable necrotising fasciitis, and another had septic arthritis and septicaemia. Two were postoperative patients in a local hospital. The other infections appeared to have been acquired in the community by local residents, of whom two had diabetes mellitus and one was on long-term corticosteroid therapy. Patients ranged in age from 46 to 68 years. Four different types of group A *Streptococcus* were isolated from blood cultures or joint aspirates from five of the infected people. A number of sporadic cases were reported from other parts of the country during the year.

Necrotising fasciitis is a rare condition in which there is extensive and rapidly progressive soft-tissue necrosis associated with fever and extreme prostration; shock and multi-organ failure are common. The need for early identification and treatment of infection in immunosuppressed patients was noted in *CMO's Update*[1].

The PHLS has begun an enhanced surveillance programme for invasive group A streptococcal infections, which will include detailed categorisation of strains and will run initially for two years.

Reference

1. Department of Health. Antibiotic therapy in immunosuppressed people. *CMO's Update* 1994; **3:** 3.

(i)   Antibiotic resistance and hospital-acquired infection

Methicillin-resistant *Staphylococcus aureus* (MRSA) has been an increasing problem in British hospitals during 1994. Epidemic strains of this organism (EMRSA) emerged in the early 1980s and new strains continue to appear. There has been a striking increase in isolations of EMRSA strain 16 since it was first identified in 1991; the number of isolates and of hospitals affected (mainly in the South-East of England) doubled during 1994. EMRSA strain 15 continues to be prevalent in the West Midlands. In September, DH gave formal support[1] to earlier clinical guidelines for control of the organism produced by the Hospital Infection Society and the British Society for Antimicrobial Chemotherapy[2].

There have been a number of prolonged hospital outbreaks of *Clostridium difficile* infection in the last few years and a DH/PHLS Working Group has produced guidance on prevention and management of the infection, which was published in September[3].

Work to revise the 1988 guidance[4] on infection control in hospitals continued during 1994. After a consultation exercise, new guidance will be issued in Spring 1995. The new guidance will take account of the re-organisation of the NHS, make recommendations to improve surveillance of hospital-acquired infection, and provide advice to purchasers and providers of health care, including independent hospitals.

References

1. NHS Executive. *Improving the effectiveness of NHS.* Heywood (Lancashire): Department of Health, 1994 (Executive Letter: EL(94)74).
2. Hospital Infection Society, British Society for Antimicrobial Chemotherapy. Revised guidelines for the control of epidemic methicillin-resistant *Staphylococcus aureus. J Hosp Infect* 1990; **16:** 351-77.
3. Department of Health. *Clostridium difficile infection: prevention and management: a report by a Department of Health/Public Health Laboratory Service Joint Working Group.* Heywood (Lancashire): Department of Health, 1994.
4. Department of Health and Social Security. *Hospital infection control: guidance on the control of infection in hospitals prepared by the Joint PHLS/DHSS Hospital Infection Working Group.* Heywood (Lancashire): Department of Health and Social Security, 1988 (Health Circular: HC(88)33).

(j)   Foodborne and waterborne diseases

Foodborne diseases

The provisional number of cases of food poisoning (formally notified and ascertained by other means) in England and Wales reported to OPCS in 1994 was 82,587 (see Table 6.9), an increase of 18% over the 69,955 cases provisionally reported in 1993[1]. *Campylobacter* continues to be the organism most commonly isolated from cases of human gastroenteritis and there was a rise in the number of reports of *Campylobacter* compared with 1993. The incidence of *Salmonella* and of verocytotoxin-producing *Escherichia coli* (VTEC) serogroup 0157 were similar to that in 1993. Listeriosis remains well below the level of the late 1980s. There was an outbreak of *Shigella sonnei* infection linked to food in 1994.

Table 6.9: *Food poisoning: reports to OPCS, England and Wales, 1982-94*

Year	Total*
1982	14253
1983	17735
1984	20702
1985	19242
1986	23948
1987	29331
1988	39713
1989	52557
1990	52145
1991	52543
1992	63347†
1993	68587‡
1994	82587**

* Statutorily notified to OPCS and ascertained by other means.
† Data for 53 reporting weeks.
‡ Confirmed cases (not provisional as used in the text).
** Provisional data.

Source: OPCS

Campylobacter enteritis

Campylobacter continues to be the most commonly isolated bacterium associated with acute gastro-enteritis in human beings. The provisional number of laboratory reports to CDSC of faecal isolation of *Campylobacter* in England and Wales during 1994 was 44,315, compared with a provisional total of 39,383 for 1993.

Salmonellosis

The number of *Salmonella* isolations reported in England and Wales and recorded on the PHLS Salmonella Data Set for 1994 was 30,428, compared with 30,650 reports in 1993 (see Table 6.10). Since 1989, the number of *Salmonella* isolations reported has been around 30,000 annually.

Table 6.10: *Salmonella in human beings, England and Wales: January to December (inclusive) 1993 and 1994*

Serotype	1993		1994	
	Total cases	Imported cases	Total cases	Imported cases
S. enteritidis				
phage type 4	17257	1282	13782	1245
other phage types	2997	498	3588	699
S. typhimurium	4778	445	5523	464
Other serotypes[1]	5618	1446	7535	1803
Total	30650	3671	30428	4211

[1] Salmonellas fully identified by the Laboratory of Enteric Pathogens (LEP) as serotypes other than *S. enteritidis* or *S. typhimurium*

Source: PHLS Salmonella Data Set

Salmonella enteritidis phage type 4 (PT4) associated with poultry and eggs is the commonest *Salmonella* to infect human beings in England and Wales. In 1994, there were 13,782 reported isolations compared with 17,258 in 1993, a 20% fall. By contrast, infection due to a multi-resistant strain of *Salmonella typhimurium* definitive type 104 (DT104) continues to increase and is now the second most prevalent *Salmonella* in human beings. Last year there were 2,117 reported isolations, compared with 1,208 in 1993. No single food source has been identified. The micro-organism is known to infect a range of food animal species, especially cattle. *Salmonella typhimurium* DT104 does not appear to be more invasive than other types of *Salmonella*. DH, the Ministry of Agriculture, Fisheries and Food (MAFF) and the PHLS continue to investigate the underlying reasons for this increase in infection.

Verocytotoxin-producing Escherichia coli (VTEC)

During 1994, the PHLS Laboratory of Enteric Pathogens identified 411 isolations of VTEC 0157 (the most common VTEC serogroup identified in cases of human illness) in England and Wales. This compares with revised figures of 385 for 1993 and of 470 for 1992. Most cases were sporadic, but some small outbreaks occurred, one of which involved visitors to a farm and contact with calves and goats. Haemolytic uraemic syndrome associated with VTEC infection continued to occur mainly in children under 10 years-of-age, with a peak between one and four years-of-age. In a number of these cases the VTEC strains belonged to serogroups other than 0157.

The first isolations of VTEC 0157 from foodstuffs in England and Wales were made from milk and beefburgers in 1993, and in 1994 there were several isolations of VTEC 0157 from foods including uncooked beefburgers, sausages and steak. The PHLS continues to monitor VTEC infection due to all serogroups.

Listeria

Isolates of *Listeria monocytogenes* received by the PHLS remained at a low level, with 112 provisionally reported in England and Wales in 1994 compared with 102 in 1993.

Foodborne outbreak of Shigella sonnei infection

In late May and early June, there was a foodborne outbreak of infection due to *Shigella sonnei*, mainly affecting adults in the South and South-West of England. Outbreaks were also reported from Scotland, Norway and Sweden. Infection appeared to be linked to the consumption of imported Spanish iceberg lettuce. Spanish authorities recommended improvements in lettuce production and food hygiene, and no foodborne outbreaks of *Shigella sonnei* occurred in the last quarter of 1994, the second main period of the year in which Spanish iceberg lettuce is imported into the UK. Food is not a commonly identified source of *Shigella sonnei* infection, and this was an unusual event.

Food surveillance has continued to increase as studies by the Advisory Committee on the Microbiological Safety of Food and the Steering Group on the Microbiological Safety of Food come into full effect.

The Steering Group on the Microbiological Safety of Food has five established working groups, one each on human epidemiology, farm animals and abattoirs, food processing, and retail catering and consumers; and a research working group to take forward a wide range of work relevant to foodborne diseases.

The human infectious intestinal disease (IID) study is now well under way but it is too soon to release data. The farm animals and abattoirs surveillance working group started surveys of VTEC in bovine faeces and of carriage rates of VTEC on beef carcasses; both will run for 12 months.

As a result of the rising incidence of *Salmonella typhimurium* DT104 in human beings and animals alike, this organism is being studied in cattle and in cereals used in animal feedstuffs.

The Food Processing Surveillance Working Group has entered the second phase of the national study of ready-to-eat meats and meat products. The group also examined warm-water prawns for a wide range of pathogens, and commissioned a survey of canneries to assess the risk posed to the consumer of canned foods. Reports of these studies should be available during 1995.

The Retail Catering and Consumer Surveillance Working Group completed three projects on potential contamination sites in catering premises; the bacteriological examination of salad items and hors d'oeuvres from self-service salad bars; and salmonella contamination in UK-produced raw chicken. The results of these completed studies should be published during 1995.

The Research Working Group published a compendium of endorsed microbiological methods for surveillance purposes, and held a symposium on foodborne viruses.

During 1994, initial steps were taken to improve overall co-ordination of microbiological food sampling, which is undertaken by a wide range of bodies including local authorities and Government bodies, the PHLS and local authority co-ordinating bodies on food and trading standards. The UK also contributes to the European Commission's (EC's) co-ordinated programme for the official control of foodstuffs, which ensures that information on various programmes of work is exchanged and allows co-ordination of sampling and of analytical methods used.

More details on the above work can be found in the Annual Report of the Steering Group on the Microbiological Safety of Food[2].

The Working Group on VTEC completed its report on the significance of VTEC as a foodborne pathogen, which will be published in 1995.

The Poultry Meat Working Group continued its extensive examination of systems used in the production of poultry meat. Its report, which will include advice on action that might reduce the incidence of foodborne pathogens in poultry meat, is expected in late 1995.

The Committee continues to identify emerging foodborne pathogens. A current area of interest is the role of viruses in foodborne disease.

Waterborne diseases

Three non-cryptosporidial waterborne outbreaks were reported in 1994 - two related to private water supplies (*Campylobacter*) and the other to inadvertent consumption of non-potable water (astrovirus). Seven outbreaks of cryptosporidiosis were reported to PHLS CDSC during the year. In only two outbreaks was drinking water considered a possible vehicle of infection. The results of a case-control study of one of these outbreaks are awaited. A group of experts has again been convened, under the chairmanship of Sir John Badenoch, to review progress in the understanding of cryptosporidiosis since publication of *Cryptosporidium in water supplies*[3] in 1990, and to produce a follow-up report.

The report of a four-year study of the health effects of sea-bathing, funded jointly by DH, the Department of the Environment, the Welsh Office and the National Rivers Authority, was submitted in January[4]. The study showed a link between indicators of faecal pollution and minor, self-limiting gastro-intestinal symptoms, but concluded that current standards for bathing water give adequate protection to health.

References

1. Department of Health. *On the State of the Public Health: the annual report of the Chief Medical Officer of the Department of Health for the year 1993*. London: Department of Health, 1994: 158-61.
2. Steering Group on the Microbiological Safety of Food. *Annual report 1993*. London: HMSO, 1994.
3. Department of Health. *Cryptosporidium in water supplies: report of the group of experts*. London: HMSO, 1990. Chair: Sir John Badenoch.
4. Department of the Environment. *Health effects of sea bathing (WMI 9021) - Phase III: Final report to the Department of the Environment: report no: DoE 3412/2*. Marlow (Buckinghamshire): WRc plc, 1994.

(k)   Travel-related disease

Health advice for travellers, the Department's free booklet that describes health risks abroad and how to avoid them, and reciprocal health care arrangements for UK residents visiting other countries, was completely revised for 1994[1]. The information is also available, and regularly updated, on the national 'Prestel' database.

Malaria

1,887 cases of imported malaria were reported to the PHLS Malaria Reference Laboratory in 1994, compared with 1,922 in 1993, 1,629 in 1992 and 2,332 in 1991. 1,176 cases (62%), mostly from West Africa, were due to the more severe *Plasmodium falciparum* infection, continuing the rising trend of recent years. There were 9 deaths. A review of malaria imported into the UK in 1992 and 1993 drew attention to the fact that over one-third of malaria cases were among settled immigrants from endemic areas who had returned to visit friends and relations[2]. Most of the people who died had not taken adequate preventive measures, but in two the diagnosis was delayed.

Hepatitis A

About 13% of cases of hepatitis A reported to the PHLS from England and Wales in 1994 included a recent history of foreign travel; the Indian subcontinent (110 cases), Africa (39) and the Mediterranean and Europe (45) were the most common destinations mentioned. A case-control study of sporadic hepatitis in England between July 1990 and June 1991 found travel abroad, particularly to the Indian subcontinent, to be the single greatest risk factor[3].

Cholera

The PHLS Laboratory of Enteric Pathogens received isolates from 17 cases of cholera imported into England and Wales in 1994. Fifteen were serogroup 01 and were associated with travel to Hong Kong (1), India (4), Pakistan (3), Thailand (2), Turkey (1), Nigeria (1) and Tunisia (3); three had travelled to more than one country. Serogroup 0139 was confirmed in two patients, one of whom had travelled to Bangladesh and Thailand and the other to Nepal and Pakistan.

Typhoid

Two hundred and one of the 227 cases of typhoid in England and Wales reported to the PHLS in 1994, including 13 family outbreaks, were associated with travel abroad - most commonly to the Indian subcontinent. 168 of 180 reported cases of paratyphoid A and 27 of 37 cases of paratyphoid B were also associated with travel abroad.

Legionnaires' disease

Seventy seven reported cases of Legionnaires' disease in England and Wales in 1994 were probably acquired abroad. Since 1987, European countries have collaborated in the surveillance of Legionnaires' disease associated with travel through the European Working Group on Legionella Infections. By the end of 1993, more than 571 cases had been reported to the scheme and more than 50 clusters (two or more cases associated with the same premises within six months) had been identified.

Other imported diseases

Laboratory reports of imported infections also included hookworm (nearly 210 reports), schistosomiasis (nearly 205), *Strongyloides*, filaria, dengue fever, jigger flea, cutaneous leishmaniasis, *Rickettsiae*, human bot fly, Tumbu fly and *Fasciola hepatica*.

References

1. UK Health Departments. *Health advice for travellers (T5)*. London: HMSO, 1994.
2. Bradley D, Warhurst D, Blaze M, Smith V. Malaria imported into the United Kingdom in 1992 and 1993. *Commun Dis Rep Rev* 1994; **13**: R169-72.
3. Maguire HC et al. A collaborative case control study of sporadic hepatitis in England. *Commun Dis Rep Rev* (in press).

CHAPTER 7

ENVIRONMENTAL HEALTH AND TOXICOLOGY

(a)   Chemical and physical agents in the environment

(i)   *Small Area Health Statistics Unit*

The Small Area Health Statistics Unit (SAHSU) is an independent academic unit based at the London School of Hygiene and Tropical Medicine. It is funded by Government to investigate claims of ill-health in the vicinity of industrial point-sources of pollution. The background and work of SAHSU has been described in previous Reports[1,2,3].

In response to claims of local cancer excesses, SAHSU has studied the incidence of cancer and mortality near to the petrochemical works at Baglan Bay, South Wales. The study was completed in 1994 and found a general excess of all cancer and of larynx cancer incidence, but this was consistent with findings for the region and not thought to be related to emissions from the plant[4]. A follow-up study of haematopoietic cancers is to be conducted near oil refineries in Great Britain.

A major study of cancer incidence near all municipal incinerators in Great Britain was also completed in 1994, covering one-fifth of the population. Despite public and scientific concerns about potentially toxic emissions from incinerators, the findings were reassuring. Nevertheless, an excess of liver cancers near the sites was considered worthy of further investigation[5].

These highly specialised investigations are made possible by the computational system developed by SAHSU based on a postcoded database of all cancer incidence; several other studies are close to completion and are expected to be published during 1995. An international workshop was held in September on the use of deprivation indices in small area studies of environment and health, with a particular emphasis on the 1991 Census. SAHSU also continues to make a major contribution to the development of statistical and computational methodology for investigating disease in small areas.

(ii)   *Air pollution*

The Committee on the Medical Effects of Air Pollutants (COMEAP) established two sub-groups in 1993 - one to advise on possible links between asthma and air pollution and the other to consider evidence about the health effects of airborne particles; after analysis of published research in these complex areas, reports are expected in late 1995. Epidemiological research on the health effects of particles is currently an area of major interest: associations between ambient concentrations of particles and a range of health indices have been shown. Much of this evidence comes from studies in North America, and the ability to detect relatively small effects depends on careful monitoring of ambient concentrations and the use of advanced statistical analysis of complex data sets[6,7]. Studies in Europe tend to confirm the results of the American studies[8,9].

In view of growing media interest and public concern about possible effects of air pollution on health, COMEAP was asked for interim advice before the sub-group's report. COMEAP endorsed the following statement, while emphasising that it may need to review the position when the sub-group has finished its work: "there appears to be sufficient evidence from studies conducted in a number of countries to give cause for concern about the possible effects of current levels of fine particles upon health. This is a complex area and it is not yet clear what role changes in low levels of particles play *vis-a-vis* changes in levels of other pollutants and temperature and humidity in causing the changes in indices of morbidity and mortality recorded in a number of studies. Despite these difficulties, which will be addressed in detail by the COMEAP sub-group on particles, reductions in levels of fine particles should be welcomed".

A major source of particles in urban areas is provided by diesel-powered motor vehicles, and COMEAP advised that, in the current state of knowledge, diesel-engined cars and light motor vehicles showed no advantage, on health grounds, over petrol-engined cars and light motor vehicles fitted with catalytic converters.

Advice from COMEAP has helped the Department of the Environment's (DoE's) Expert Panel on Air Quality Standards (EPAQS) to recommend ambient air quality standards for the United Kingdom (UK). During 1994, EPAQS published four recommendations for air quality standards (ppb = parts per billion; ppm = parts per million):

- benzene: 5 ppb measured as a running annual average;

- ozone: 50 ppb measured as a running 8-hour average;

- 1,3-butadiene: 1 ppb measured as a running annual average; *and*

- carbon monoxide: 10 ppm measured as a running 8-hour average.

EPAQS is currently considering a standard for sulphur dioxide and is working closely with COMEAP to make a recommendation on airborne particles.

Air pollution research is a priority within the Department of Health's (DH's) centrally commissioned research programme and important areas of research were identified by discussion with expert advisory groups. The Department, together with DoE and the Medical Research Council (MRC), issued a call in October for research proposals on air pollution and respiratory disease. The Institute for Environment and Health (IEH) at Leicester managed the initial consideration of research proposals arising from this request, and the co-ordinated research programme will eventually award £5 million for research contracts.

(iii)   Institute for Environment and Health

The MRC's Institute for Environment and Health, which is supported by funding from the DoE and DH, produced two reports in 1994[10,11]. The first, *Air pollution and health: understanding the uncertainties*[10], based on an international workshop in collaboration with the World Health Organization (WHO), formed a major contribution to the Second European Conference on Environment and Health. The second report, *Air pollution and respiratory disease: UK research priorities*[11] was based on a UK expert workshop on possible linkages between exposure to environmental chemicals and respiratory disease. DH is working in collaboration with DoE and the MRC to support a coherent programme of research on possible health effects of air pollution, focused on Government priorities. The call for research proposals was managed by the IEH, which also held an international workshop on air quality in the home.

(iv)   Committee on Medical Aspects of Radiation in the Environment

The Committee on Medical Aspects of Radiation in the Environment (COMARE) continued to fulfil its remit "to assess and advise Government on the health effects of natural and man-made radiation in the environment and to assess the adequacy of the available data and the need for further research".

Specifically, COMARE issued a statement regarding the raised incidence of certain childhood cancers near Dounreay, Scotland[12]. Work on the incidence of childhood cancer around nuclear installations has continued since the publication of the 1984 report[13] of the Black Advisory Group regarding the incidence of cancer in young people in the vicinity of Sellafield in West Cumbria; a further report should be published during 1996.

(v)   Environment and health

The European Regional Office of the WHO, in collaboration with the European Community (EC), organised the second Ministerial Conference on Environment and Health at Helsinki in June, which was attended by Ministers from over 50 countries which now fall within the WHO European Region; in many cases, including the UK and most EC countries, health and environment Ministers attended. The main background papers for the conference described 'Concern for Europe's Tomorrow' - about environmental and associated health issues in Europe; a draft environmental health action plan for Europe (EHAPE) set broad objectives and priorities for action both at European and national levels.

The principal outcomes of the Conference were wide commitment to EHAPE and to the development of national environmental health action plans (NEHAPs); and a decision to establish a European Environment and Health Committee (EEHC) to oversee and assist with the development of NEHAPs and to address common and transboundary environment and health issues.

The UK was an active participant in preparations for the Conference and at the meeting itself. Since the Helsinki meeting, UK has agreed to become one of the countries to develop pilot NEHAPs and is scheduled to produce an action plan by early 1996; the UK was also nominated as a member of the EEHC and has offered to host the Third European Conference in 1999.

At the international conference on chemical safety (ICCS) held in Stockholm during April, delegates from over 100 countries agreed to establish an Inter-Governmental Forum on Chemical Safety (IGFCS). The conference, and the establishment of the Forum, implement one of the commitments entered into by the Government when it endorsed Agenda 21, the international action plan agreed at the United Nations (UN) Conference on Environment and Development (the 'Rio Summit') in June 1992. Chapter 19 of Agenda 21 is concerned with the environmentally sound management of toxic chemicals and identified six programme areas for priority work. The Forum is a non-institutional body that operates by consensus among the Governmental representatives from 31 countries. Its main purpose is to develop strategies to implement Chapter 19 of Agenda 21, and specifically to achieve the targets set at Stockholm for the six priority programme areas identified at the Rio Summit. Further meetings of this Forum are planned for 1997 and 2000 and the interim work will be carried forward by the Forum Bureau, with an Inter-Sessional Group (ISG) which will meet annually. DH has set up an Inter-Departmental Co-ordination Group to consider UK input into this area.

(vi)   *Surveillance of diseases possibly due to non-infectious environmental hazards*

The Abrams Committee[14] recommended that DH should set up an expert Working Group to consider whether, and if so which, diseases might be appropriate for surveillance with regard to non-infectious environmental hazards.

The Group has reported to the Chief Medical Officer and the Department is considering its suggestions. The main conclusions and recommendations were that:

-    with the exception of certain agents associated with cancer (eg, asbestos with mesothelioma), the Group was unable to identify any diseases which were known to be principally caused by single environmental factors;

-    it was important to recognise that surveillance could be used to raise questions for further investigation;

-    trends in diseases of current concern, such as asthma, may or may not be related to environmental hazards. It is known that asthma attacks can be provoked by environmental factors such as high levels of air pollution. The Group recommended that, in the first instance, efforts should be concentrated on meaningful surveillance of asthma and acute respiratory responses;

- a series of inter-related pilot surveys to examine the feasibility of more routine surveillance of asthma and other respiratory diseases should be set up at the local level. The scope for greater use of existing databases - for example, morbidity and research reports by GPs, and Prescription Pricing Authority and hospital admissions data - should be investigated; *and*

- surveillance of clusters of cancer and congenital abnormalities should be a priority; arrangements already exist for investigation of health statistics in small areas, through SAHSU, and this work may soon be augmented by the Office of Population Censuses and Surveys (OPCS). It was recognised that data quality was often a limiting factor and the Group recommended better and more timely data on cancer incidence and congenital abnormalities for surveillance purposes.

References

1. Department of Health. *On the State of Public Health: the annual report of the Chief Medical Officer of the Department of Health for the year 1991.* London: HMSO, 1992; 152.
2. Department of Health. *On the State of Public Health: the annual report of the Chief Medical Officer of the Department of Health for the year 1992.* London: HMSO,1993; 172.
3. Department of Health. *On the State of Public Health: the annual report of the Chief Medical Officer of the Department of Health for the year 1993.* London: HMSO, 1994; 164.
4. Sans S, Elliott P, Kleinschmidt I, et al. Cancer incidence and mortality near the Baglan Bay petrochemical works, South Wales. *Occup Environ Med* (in press).
5. Elliott P, Shaddick G, Kleinschmidt I, et al. Cancer incidence near municipal solid waste incinerators in Great Britain. *Br J Cancer* (in press).
6. Dockery DW, Pope CA III. Acute respiratory effects of particulate air pollution. *Annu Rev Publ Health* 1994; **15:** 107-32.
7. Schwartz J. Air pollution and hospital admissions for the elderly in Detroit, Michigan. *Am J Respir Crit Care Med* 1994; **150:** 648-55.
8. Walters S, Griffiths RK, Ayres JG. Temporal association between hospital admissions for asthma in Birmingham and ambient levels of sulphur dioxide and smoke. *Thorax* 1994; **49:** 133-40.
9. Studnicka MJ, Frischer T, Meinert R, et al. Acidic particles and lung function in children: a summer camp study in the Austrian Alps. *Am J Respir Crit Care Med* (in press).
10. Medical Research Council Institute for Environment and Health. *Air pollution and health: understanding the uncertainties.* Norwich: Institute for Environment and Health, 1994.
11. Medical Research Council Institute for Environment and Health. *Air pollution and respiratory disease: UK research priorities.* Norwich: Institute for Environment and Health, 1994.
12. House of Commons. Parliamentary Debate. Childhood Cancer, Dounreay. *Hansard* 19 July 1994; **247:** Col 120-1.
13. Department of Health. *Investigation of the possible increased incidence of cancer in West Cumbria: report of the Independent Advisory Group.* London: HMSO, 1984. Chair: Sir Douglas Black.
14. Department of Health. *Public health responsibilities of the NHS and roles of others.* Heywood (Lancashire): Department of Health, 1993 (Miscellaneous Circular: MISC(93)56).

(b)   Toxicological safety

(i)   *Food chemical hazards*

During 1994, DH published new guidelines on the management of outbreaks of foodborne illness[1]. The new guidance is designed "to be of assistance to all those from a variety of disciplines who may be involved in an outbreak of foodborne illness". While most outbreaks of foodborne illness tend to be associated with bacterial contamination, it is now well recognised that some outbreaks may be due to chemical contamination of food. Thus, in addition to the handling of bacterial incidents, the management guide sets out requirements for handling incidents caused by chemical contamination.

DH only becomes directly involved in the management of local outbreaks due to chemical contamination in exceptional circumstances, but has an important advisory role to Ministers. Its medical and scientific staff, in conjunction with Environmental Health Officers and colleagues in the Ministry of Agriculture, Fisheries and Food (MAFF) can provide expert and definitive advice on most incidents, but an enormous number of chemicals have the potential to contaminate food and the range of expertise necessary to deal with questions on toxicity is vast.

For public health officials with limited experience of chemical contamination of food, the guide offers advice on the membership of outbreak control groups. A list of foodborne illnesses caused by chemicals, as a guide to the wide variety of ways that poisoning episodes can present, points out the ease with which such symptoms can be confused with those caused by bacterial contamination.

(ii)   *Food chemical prioritisation*

The Committee on Carcinogenicity of Chemicals in Food, Consumer Products and the Environment (COC) agreed a scheme to assign relative priorities to carcinogenic chemicals found in food. This prioritisation is based on an assessment of hazard (using all relevant human and animal data), and on the extent and distribution of exposure to the chemical in question. A measure of carcinogenic potency may be included for particular categories of chemicals (such as genotoxic carcinogens). This scheme will be a useful guide to help to focus official attention and resources where they are most needed.

(iii)   *Peanut anaphylaxis*

There are no definitive figures available as to how many people in the UK are in danger of anaphylactic reactions to nuts, but deaths from peanut anaphylaxis have highlighted the importance of this issue. DH's Health Aspects of the Environment and Food Division liaises with colleagues in MAFF's Food Safety Directorate to ensure that voluntary labelling of food packaging specifies all nuts, including groundnuts and tree and sesame nuts, to allow consumers to exercise choice when purchasing food. DH also assists MAFF in issuing advice to consumers to make them more aware of potential risks[2] and has informed the medical profession about recent developments[3].

(iv)   *Traditional remedies*

Attention was drawn to the possible adverse reactions to traditional remedies by an article in *CMO's Update* in November[4]. Clinicians should be aware that their patients may be taking traditional remedies (whether licensed or unlicensed) in addition to allopathic medicines, and that unusual adverse reactions may develop. The results of research undertaken at Guy's Hospital Poisons Unit, and funded by MAFF, on adverse reactions to these remedies has now been published[5].

The Committee on Toxicity of Chemicals in Food, Consumer Products and the Environment (COT) examined these data at its meeting in June. COT was sufficiently concerned to issue advice which went to the Food Advisory Committee (FAC) and was considered by FAC at its meeting in September. FAC discussed a number of courses of action: in view of the complexity of this issue, it asked officials to report back to the Committee after they had spoken to and canvassed the opinion of a wide range of interested parties before recommending any detailed action.

(v)   The Advisory Committee on Novel Foods and Processes

The Advisory Committee on Novel Foods and Processes (ACNFP) is an independent committee of experts appointed by Ministers to advise on any matters relating to novel foods or foods produced by use of novel processes. DH provides part of the secretariat to the Committee, covering particularly medical, toxicological and nutritional safety aspects.

Food technology progresses quickly: many new foods or food components that the Committee is asked to assess might have the potential to affect a person's health. Fat replacers may affect the absorption of fat-soluble vitamins or may affect thrombogenesis by altering the balance of lipids in the body, and foods intended to influence bowel microflora may also have effects on digestion and drug absorption. Safety assessments of novel foods must take all these aspects into consideration.

(vi)   Genetically modified food plants

In 1994, the ACNFP considered the food safety aspects of products derived from three genetically modified (GM) plants - tomato paste from GM tomatoes, oil from GM oilseed rape and processed food products from GM soya beans.

The Committee compared nutritional and toxicological equivalence of food products derived from the GM plants and from their conventional counterparts, and reviewed the genetic modification procedures used to produce the GM plants and the possibility of untoward secondary effects.

ACNFP was satisfied that the GM plants, and food products derived therefrom, were substantially equivalent to their conventional counterparts. However, as there is little experience in predicting the effect of genetic drift on the metabolism of any plant, the Committee asked that appropriate data be provided, at regular intervals, to confirm the long-term stability of GM plants.

(vii)   Fat replacers

Variations in the intake of dietary fats may affect factors involved in thrombogenesis. During its assessment of a synthetic triglyceride intended for use in confectionery as a replacement for cocoa butter, the ACNFP discussed the general assessment of novel fats for possible thrombotic effects. This discussion highlighted various aspects of the nutritional toxicology of novel foods, where nutritional safety as opposed to nutritional adequacy is a key issue. The Committee agreed that studies to assess the effects on thrombotic potential may be required for certain novel fats.

(viii)   Man-made mineral fibres

The COC provided the Health and Safety Executive (HSE) with an update of previous advice[6] on man-made mineral fibre used in domestic insulation (ie, glass fibres, rock-wool and slag-wool). Evidence of lung cancer in occupational studies with confounding factors was documented during earlier technological phases. However, no evidence of lung cancer has been documented under modern working conditions, and these fibres were not carcinogenic in studies in which rats were exposed to high concentrations of respirable fibres, and thus should not be classified as carcinogens under the criteria of the Dangerous Substances Directive (67/548/EEC). Nevertheless, as some doubts remain, COC recommended that there should be continued monitoring of workers and agreed that it would be prudent to maintain existing controls. Further epidemiological data should become available in 1995.

(ix)   Organization for Economic Co-operation and Development guidelines for testing chemicals for toxicity

The Organization for Economic Co-operation and Development (OECD) guidelines play a key role in international harmonisation of methods to investigate the toxicity of chemicals and help to avoid needless duplication of studies with minor variations for authorities in different countries. DH represents the UK in negotiations to update these guidelines to take account of animal welfare considerations, as well as advances in science. This work is facilitated by a Toxicology Shadow Group, which allows consultation with other Government Departments, researchers and industry.

Considerable progress was made in 1994. Following a UK initiative, a revised guideline for the 28-day repeated-dose oral toxicity study was adopted, which will enhance the ability to detect compounds with neurotoxic and immunotoxic potential, or effects on reproductive organs, without the use of more animals.

Initial proposals for genetic toxicology guidelines were considered at a consultation meeting hosted by DH in 1992; extensive discussions to seek consensus followed, culminating in an OECD meeting of national nominated experts in Rome, chaired by DH. Agreement was reached on updating seven existing guidelines and on one new guideline; these recommendations should be formally adopted in 1995.

(x)   Pesticides

The approval and review of pesticides is the responsibility of six Government Departments, including DH, and Ministers are advised by the Advisory Committee on Pesticides (ACP) - a body of independent experts. The ACP has a review programme for existing approvals for pesticides[7], and during the year one of those considered was lindane. The uses of lindane have been reviewed on a number of occasions, and the latest review is focusing on the use of lindane on arable crops; it will be concluded early in 1995.

New regulations to set out permitted maximum residue levels (MRLs) of pesticides in food were approved by Parliament in 1994[8]; these regulations made changes in the 1988 UK regulations[9], increasing the number of crop/pesticide combinations covered, and also implemented MRLs set by the EC.

The 1993 annual report of the Working Party on Pesticide Residues was published in November[10], and describes the results of surveillance monitoring of food for pesticide residues. Sampling is split between UK-produced and imported food in approximate proportion to their respective contributions to the UK diet. Breaches of MRLs only occurred in a small proportion of crops, but MRLs which were exceeded included disulfoton and phorate in carrots and dithiocarbamates in lettuce from the UK. In imported food, breaches were seen for dithiocarbamates in French beans and bromide in rice. Residues of organochlorine pesticides were seen in imported lamb and rabbits. None of these breaches was thought likely to be of health concern, but appropriate action is being taken to prevent recurrence.

(xi)   Veterinary drugs

Sheep dips are insecticidal mixtures used to treat ectoparasitic diseases of sheep, particularly sheep scab. Organochlorine sheep dips were phased out in 1985 because of their biopersistence. Most current sheep dips contain organophosphates (OPs), which are powerful anticholinesterases[11]. Sheep dips are veterinary medicines licensed under the Medicines Act 1968[12]. MAFF and DH Ministers constitute the Licensing Authority and act after advice from the Veterinary Products Committee (VPC).

In 1991, reports started to circulate that farmers dipping sheep were experiencing various symptoms that could broadly be divided into two groups: acute (consisting of a transient influenza-like illness), and long-term (more varied but including poor memory, depression, headache, pyrexia and sometimes signs referable to the peripheral nervous system). Because of concern about OP sheep dips, the VPC reviewed sheep dips twice during 1993, and decided existing licences should remain in force. However, because of evidence that adequate precautions were not being observed during dipping, the VPC decided that a Certificate of Competence should be held by those wishing to use OP sheep dips. This requirement is being enforced at point of sale by Regulations[13] made under the Medicines Act 1968[12]; these came into force in April and require that a Certificate of Enrolment for the Certificate of Competence is necessary before OP sheep dips can be sold or supplied by a registered agricultural merchant. The same Regulations will require the sheep dipper to have the Certificate of Competence (as opposed to just having enrolled) by April 1995. In addition to the Certificate of Competence, the VPC set up an Expert Panel to consider long-term effects of OPs on sheep dippers and any research that might be helpful. The Panel met on several occasions and tenders have been invited to fulfil the Panel's main research recommendation for an epidemiological survey. DH will partly fund this work.

EC Regulations for the authorisation and supervision of medicines for human and veterinary use have been made[14].

References

1. Department of Health. *Management of outbreaks of foodborne illness.* London: Department of Health, 1994.
2. Ministry of Agriculture, Fisheries and Food. *Food allergy and other unpleasant reactions to food.* London: Ministry of Agriculture, Fisheries and Food, 1994.
3. Department of Health. Peanut anaphylaxis. *CMO's Update* 1994; **2**: 5.
4. Department of Health. Adverse reactions to alternative remedies. *CMO's Update* 1994; **4**: 2.
5. Perharic L, Shaw D, Colbridge M, House I, Leon C, Murray V. Toxicological problems resulting from exposure to traditional remedies and food supplements. *Drug Safety* 1994; **11**: 284-94.
6. Department of Health and Social Security. *On the State of the Public Health: the annual report of the Chief Medical Officer of the Department of Health and Social Security for the year 1987.* London: HMSO, 1988; 100-2.
7. Ministry of Agriculture, Fisheries and Food Advisory Committee on Pesticides. *Advisory Committee on Pesticides Annual Report (1994).* London: HMSO, 1994.
8. *Pesticides (Maximum Residue Levels in Crops, Food and Feeding Stuffs) Regulations 1994.* London: HMSO, 1994 (Statutory Instrument: SI 1994 no. 1985).
9. *Pesticides (Maximum Residue Levels in Food) Regulations 1988.* London: HMSO, 1988 (Statutory Instrument: SI 1988 no. 1378).
10. Ministry of Agriculture, Fisheries and Food, Health and Safety Executive. *Annual Report of the Working Party on Pesticide Residues 1993.* London: HMSO (in press).
11. Marrs TC. Organophosphate poisoning. *Pharmacol Therapeut* 1993; **58**: 51-66.
12. *Medicines Act 1968.* London: HMSO, 1968.
13. *The Medicines (Veterinary Drugs) (Pharmacy and Merchants' List) (Amendment) Order 1994.* London: HMSO, 1994 (Statutory Instrument: SI 1994 no. 599).
14. Council Regulation (EEC) no. 2309/93 of 22 July 1993. *Off J Eur Commun* 1993; **L214**: 1-21.

CHAPTER 8

MEDICAL EDUCATION, TRAINING AND STAFFING

(a)   Junior doctors' hours

In 1991, the 'New Deal'[1] introduced a timetable to reduce junior doctors' hours through the use of new working arrangements and explicit limits on contracted and actual hours of duty. Virtually all posts contracted for a maximum average over 83 hours per week had been eliminated by the end of 1993. During 1994, the Department of Health's (DH's) main aim was to eliminate hard-pressed on-call posts contracted for more than 72 hours per week. By 31 December, 1,793 such posts remained, a fall of 72.5% in nine months. Tackling these hard-pressed posts remain a priority.

DH continues to support the 'New Deal' with central funds. Between 1991 and September 1994, 687 extra consultant and 163 additional staff grade posts were created expressly to help to reduce junior doctors' hours, at a cost of £49 million in 1994/95. Regional Health Authorities (RHAs) also developed many local projects, including part-funded consultant posts, more nursing and support workers, and further improvements in living conditions.

Following the Minister for Health's re-affirmation, at the outset of the year, of the Government's continuing commitment to the 'New Deal', further staff grade posts were released up to the 10% national ceiling and Regional Task Forces, in consultation with postgraduate deans, were able to vary the number of senior house officer (SHO) posts within Regions. This controlled staffing expansion has produced a further 845 medical posts funded locally.

Regional Task Forces are also using a range of other measures to meet current targets, including new working patterns, improved team working and cross-cover, more effective use of skill-mix across all hospital grades, and redistribution of posts between specialties or sites.

Levels of work intensity within overall contracted hours are also now being scrutinised - a process which involves co-operation with junior doctors themselves to ensure that actual hours of work are accurately monitored. Regional Task Forces have been asked to prepare comparative data to show local progress on all aspects of the 'New Deal'.

Reference

1.   Department of Health. *Hours of work of doctors in training: the new deal.* London: Department of Health, 1991 (Executive Letter: EL(91)82).

(b) 'Achieving a Balance' and the Advisory Group on Medical and Dental Education, Training and Staffing

Achieving a Balance: plan for action[1], published in 1987, is a ten-year plan aimed at improving patient care, primarily by increasing the proportion of care provided by consultants via an annual increase of at least 2% in consultant numbers. In practice, this suggested expansion rate has been exceeded, averaging 2.9% (in whole-time equivalent consultant posts) annually between 1989 and 1994 when the effects of centrally-funded initiatives, such as posts established to help to reduce junior doctors' hours, are taken into account.

Ministers' acceptance of the recommendations of *Hospital Doctors: training for the future*[2] (the Calman report) had considerable implications for the work of the Joint Planning Advisory Committee (JPAC). The National Health Service (NHS) Executive felt that it would be inappropriate for JPAC to continue to issue quotas based on the old senior registrar and career registrar structures when DH policy was moving in another direction. However, workforce planning controls had to be maintained and for this reason only the activities of JPAC were suspended early in 1994; the quotas which were in place at the time of the suspension remain in force.

Advisory machinery for medical and dental staffing has developed in an incremental way since *Achieving a Balance*[1] was first agreed and published, leading to overlapping committee structures and responsibilities. It became clear that a single body was needed to oversee all workforce issues, supported by a simplified and streamlined advisory structure. The new system will accommodate recent developments, including:

- the introduction of NHS Trusts, which has led to a much larger number of employing bodies for career grade doctors;

- proposed changes in the central management of the NHS involving the abolition of RHAs and their replacement by a smaller number of Regional Offices, with concomitant changes in the management of specialist training;

- changes in the delivery of medical and dental education and training, in particular those outlined in *Hospital Doctors: training for the future*[2], recently accepted by the Government; *and*

- the 'New Deal' on junior doctors' hours[3], and the identification of changes needed in existing manpower controls to deliver targets for December 1994.

During 1994, Ministers approved the establishment of a new Advisory Group on Medical and Dental Education, Training and Staffing, (AGMETS). The Group, chaired by the Chief Medical Officer, first met on 7 December 1994, and its membership includes: representatives of junior and senior doctors (from the

Junior Doctors' Committee, the Joint Consultants' Committee, the Central Consultants and Specialists' Committee, and the General Medical Services Committee of the British Medical Association, the medical Royal Colleges and other groups); representatives from purchasers and providers of healthcare; and NHS Executive staff (including the director of human resources and the medical director). One of AGMETS' major tasks is to provide advice to the NHS Executive, through a sub-group, the Specialist Workforce Advisory Group, on the numbers of doctors in higher specialist training. The new arrangements should facilitate the introduction of the recommendations of the Calman report[2]. The key features of the new planning process differ markedly from, and replace, those of the old JPAC mechanism.

References

1. Newton T, Grabham AH, Roberts G. *Hospital Medical Staffing: Achieving a Balance: plan for action: a report issued by the steering group for implementation on behalf of the Health Departments, the Joint Consultants Committee and the Chairmen of Regional Health Authorities.* London: Department of Health and Social Security, 1987.
2. Department of Health. *Hospital Doctors: training for the future: the report of the working group on specialist medical training.* London: Department of Health, 1993. Chair: Dr Kenneth Calman.
3. Department of Health. *Hours of work of doctors in training: the new deal.* London: Department of Health, 1991 (Executive Letter: EL(91)82).

(c)   Medical Manpower Standing Advisory Committee

The Medical Manpower Standing Advisory Committee (MMSAC)[1], to become the Medical Workforce Standing Advisory Committee in January 1995, is due to publish its second report in Summer 1995. The report is expected to recommend that more doctors need to be trained in the United Kingdom (UK). Recommendations will take account of cost implications and the capacity of medical schools, and are likely to take the form of a gradual increase in medical school intake for five years from 1996 to arrive at a maximum annual target intake of 4,970 by the year 2000, with no change to the current overseas student quota of 7.5% of total intake. The Committee is also expected to address key issues that affect medical workforce planning including advances in medical technology, management and medical audit skills of doctors, and changes to the skill mix between health care professionals.

Reference

1. Department of Health. *Planning the medical workforce: Medical Manpower Standing Advisory Committee: first report.* London: Department of Health, 1992.

(d)   Equal opportunities for doctors

Equality of opportunity remains an important priority within the NHS. Initiatives arising from implementation of the 'New Deal' on junior doctors hours[1] and the Calman report[2] will shape the future of higher specialist training for doctors, and are likely to make training for hospital practice more attractive to young doctors who have family commitments. The introduction of a new grade for higher specialist trainees will require a revision of the arrangements for flexible training, and should provide the opportunity to make flexible training an integral part of this new grade from the outset.

Goal 3 of Opportunity 2000[3], to increase the percentage of women consultants from 15.5% in 1991 to 20% by 1994, was not achieved: this very challenging target was set within a short timescale. Figures from September 1993 indicate that women comprised about 18% of the total consultant workforce.

There has been a steady increase in the number of doctors in flexible training. The career registrar scheme has been very successful, and in December 1994 there were 370 doctors training flexibly at this grade - an increase of more than 165 since the beginning of 1993, and an increase of 80 during the year. The £5.8 million held centrally to fund this scheme will be included in RHAs' baseline allocations from April 1995.

The senior registrar scheme has played an important part in promoting flexible working for women doctors. Of the 574 approved posts allocated across all specialties, some 445 were in use in October 1994 - an increase of 11% on last year. Administrative arrangements governing the timetable for the annual competition to enter the scheme were felt to be too restrictive and, for the 1994/95 competition, the closing date for applications was at the discretion of postgraduate deans.

In July, the Women in Surgical Training (WIST) scheme arranged a seminar for women in flexible training; the programme included addresses by a part-time consultant surgeon, a trainee surgeon, an associate postgraduate dean, and representatives of the Joint Committee on Higher Specialist Training and DH. A third WIST conference is planned for June 1995.

A new Working Group of deans, associate deans and representatives of medical Royal Colleges, met three times during 1994 to share ideas and information about equal opportunities and flexible training.

References

1. Department of Health. *Hours of work of doctors in training: the new deal.* London: Department of Health, 1991 (Executive Letter: EL(91)82).
2. Department of Health. *Hospital doctors: training for the future: the report of the working group on specialist medical training.* London: Department of Health, 1993. Chair: Dr Kenneth Calman.
3. Department of Health. *Women in the NHS: an implementation guide to Opportunity 2000.* London: Department of Health, 1992.

(e)   Part-time consultants scheme

The part-time consultant scheme, begun in 1993[1], provided pump-priming central funding to stimulate the creation of new, part-time consultant posts to prevent the loss of highly skilled medical staff whose individual circumstances did not allow them to take up a full-time appointment. This scheme included senior registrars who had successfully completed part-time training.

A second tranche of 85 new posts was announced in April[2]: nearly 500 bids had been received from employing bodies, and these were carefully assessed against a range of objective criteria. The approved new posts were spread across the whole range of medical specialties and across the RHAs. The successful bidders were notified in early August, and the new consultants began to take up their posts towards the end of the year. Central funding for the posts will continue until March 1997, after which funding should be secured through purchaser contracts in the normal way. It is hoped that the success of this scheme will encourage employers to experiment increasingly with flexible working patterns to ensure staff satisfaction whilst still providing high quality health care for patients.

References

1. Department of Health. *Medical and dental staffing: part-time consultants.* Heywood (Lancashire): Department of Health, 1993 (Executive Letter: EL(93)39).
2. Department of Health. *Medical and dental staffing: centrally funded part-time consultants scheme.* Heywood (Lancashire): Department of Health, 1994 (Executive Letter: EL(94)42).

(f)   New career structure for doctors in child health

Guidance on the new career structure and integration procedures for doctors in child health was issued in March[1]. This included arrangements for the assimilation of clinical and senior clinical medical officers into the hospital staffing structure as part of a combined child health service. The guidance set out the procedures for re-grading, if doctors wished to apply for it, with applications under the scheme to be made to the employer by March 1995.

Reference

1. Department of Health. *Assimilation of Senior Clinical Medical Officers and Clinical Medical Officers into a combined child health service.* Heywood (Lancashire): Department of Health, 1994 (Health Service Guidelines: HSG(94)10).

(g)   Postgraduate, continuing and specialist medical education

In December 1993, the Minister for Health announced[1] that the Government had accepted in full the recommendations of the report of the Working Group on Specialist Medical Training (the Calman report)[2]. Implementation of the report's recommendations would result in shorter, better structured and more intensive training for doctors, who would complete their specialist training earlier; patients should also benefit as more care would be provided by doctors who had completed their specialist training. A key recommendation of the report was the introduction of a new unified training grade, replacing existing registrar and senior registrar grades, to reduce delays in progress through training and to enable the introduction of a better planned and seamless training structure.

A working party was set up in the Spring to develop a framework for the operation of these recommendations, including entry to, progress through, and exit from the new grade; it also addressed the transitional arrangements that would be required. Clear curricula on which to base new training programmes are essential and the medical Royal Colleges have made substantial progress in the development of an educational framework for the new grade.

The initial report on specialist medical training did not address the needs of three important groups of trainee doctors: doctors from overseas; those wishing to pursue academic and research medicine; and those training in general practice. Three further working groups were convened to give particular consideration to their needs: their reports will reflect a careful analysis of complex and evolving training arrangements, and any recommendations, if accepted, will be taken into account when planning future provisions for postgraduate education.

Work was also taken forward, in close partnership with the General Medical Council (GMC) and medical Royal Colleges, on the legislative and practical arrangements for the introduction of a Certificate of Completion of Specialist Training (CCST). The CCST will define unambiguously the end-point of specialist training to comply with the European Community's (EC's) Directive on Specialist Medical Training and to safeguard standards of training in the UK. A range of complex issues was considered, including the arrangements for a Competent Authority which under EC law would have specific responsibilities for specialist training.

Substantial progress was also made on the development of a national information strategy to support workforce planning, postgraduate education and research in the NHS[3]. This strategy is based on the introduction of a Regional and specialty-specific national training number, required by all trainees who participate in higher specialist training programmes. A separate national programme/post number would record the current educational status of any training programme or post.

Discussions to identify optimum arrangements for postgraduate medical and dental education in the light of changes in the NHS management structure continued throughout the year; the important management role of deans was emphasised. It was decided during the year that the interim arrangements for funding medical training grade posts would continue for the time being, with postgraduate deans holding 50% of the basic salary costs for all trainees. Long-term arrangements are still under consideration.

In June, a national conference was held to launch a consultation document on continuing medical education (CME), to ensure a coherent and affordable national strategy. At the end of the year, responses to this consultation exercise were still under consideration. A number of medical Royal Colleges launched their own CME initiatives in 1994 to encourage consultants and other career-grade specialists to pursue relevant and effective programmes of CME.

References

1. Department of Health. *Minister endorses measures to tackle shortfall of doctors in 21st century.* London: Department of Health, 1993 (Press release: H93/710).

2. Department of Health. *Hospital Doctors: training for the future: the report of the working group on specialist medical training*. London: Department of Health, 1993. Chair: Dr Kenneth Calman.
3. NHS Executive, National Training Number Implementation Steering Committee. *Guidance on introducing national training, post and programme numbers: a report to the NHS Executive Medical Education, Training and Staffing Division, Health Care Directorate*. Leeds: Department of Health, 1994.

(h)   Medical (Professional Performance) Bill

In 1992, the GMC put forward proposals[1] that would enable it to address complaints about doctors whose standard of professional performance was deficient in circumstances where the matter was not covered by its existing health and conduct procedures. The GMC consulted on its proposals[1] and received widespread support for them from within the medical profession and outside. The GMC then approached the Department to see if it would support legislation to implement its proposals. Subsequently, in November 1994, the Government announced its intention[2] to seek Parliamentary approval for the necessary amendments to the Medical Act 1983[3].

The primary aim of the procedures proposed by the GMC is to protect the public. In relevant cases the procedures would include an assessment of a doctor's standards of professional performance. If considered deficient on assessment, a doctor would be advised to remedy such deficiencies through, for example, remedial training, and it is envisaged that most doctors would be co-operative. Nevertheless, it is also recognised that some doctors would either not wish or not be able to improve their performance, and in some such circumstances it is proposed that sanctions could be taken against a doctor, including suspension of or imposed conditions on his or her registration.

References

1. General Medical Council. *Proposed changes to the Medical Act 1983 to improve the working of the GMC's conduct and health procedures*. London: General Medical Council, 1992.
2. House of Commons. Parliamentary Debate. Debate on the Address (Department of Health). *Hansard* 16 November 1994; **250**: Col 34.
3. *Medical Act 1983*. London: HMSO, 1983.

(i)   Undergraduate medical and dental education

In December 1993, the GMC published its report on undergraduate medical education[1]. *Tomorrow's doctors* seeks to match medical education to developments in medical practice and the changing patterns of health care delivery, with suggestions for radical change in medical school curricula to be introduced over the next five years.

In 1993, DH set up a scheme to help English medical schools to implement the proposed curriculum changes. The programme involved centrally funded expenditure of £1.2 million in 1994/95; a further £1.27 million will be provided in 1995/96 and the initiative has now been extended until September 1998. The programme covers all medical schools in England and last year was extended to cover dental schools; similar initiatives have also been launched in Scotland, Wales and Northern Ireland. Each school is required to appoint a 'facilitator' to submit reports on progress to the Department; feedback so far has been encouraging. The scheme has generated considerable enthusiasm and commitment to change, and most schools now have a clear timetable for implementation of many of the suggested changes.

The financing of clinical facilities provided by NHS Trusts to undergraduate medical and dental students has also been reviewed, partly because of planned changes in the funding of clinical research and partly because of reforms to the regional management of the NHS. Ministers therefore decided to set up a review of arrangements for the Service Increment for Teaching and Research (SIFTR) to be completed during 1995.

Reference

1.   General Medical Council. *Tomorrow's doctors: recommendations on undergraduate medical education.* London: General Medical Council, 1993.

(j)   Doctors' performance

An examination of this complex subject was commissioned in September 1993 by the Secretary of State for Health from the Chief Medical Officer "to review current guidance and procedures relating to doctors whose performance appears to fall below acceptable standards", after concerns were raised within the medical profession and by NHS management that the procedures and mechanisms for dealing with poor performance by medical practitioners are confusing and possibly inadequate. During 1994, the Review Group, which included doctors, NHS managers and a patients' representative, considered current guidance available to the NHS and other employers of doctors and took evidence from medical professionals, medical defence organisations, employers and consumer interests[1].

Reference

1.   Department of Health. *Maintaining medical excellence: review of guidance on doctors' performance.* Leeds: NHS Executive (in press).

(k)   Locum doctors

The Working Group set up in December 1993 to examine ways to improve quality control in relation to locum doctors working in the NHS reported in November[1]. Its report contains recommendations designed to reduce the dependence of hospitals on locum doctors and to improve quality control procedures in the short and the long term, and a code of practice for locum appointments is proposed. It is expected that a document will be published early in 1995 for a period of consultation with interested bodies.

Reference

1.   Department of Health. *Hospital locum doctors: the report of the Locums Working Group: a consultative document.* Leeds: NHS Executive, 1994.

CHAPTER 9

OTHER TOPICS OF INTEREST IN 1994

(a)   Medicines Control Agency

(i)   Role and performance

The Medicines Control Agency (MCA) is an executive agency which reports through its Chief Executive, Dr Keith Jones, to the Secretary of State for Health. Its role is to advise Ministers and to protect public health through the control of human medicines, and its primary concern is that medicines available to the public should meet the most stringent criteria for safety, efficacy and quality.

On behalf of Health Ministers (the Licensing Authority), the MCA approves medicines for marketing through the provision of a licence, monitors medicines after licensing, takes action to resolve drug safety concerns and carries out inspection and enforcement under the provisions of the Medicines Act 1968[1], associated United Kingdom (UK) legislation and relevant European Community (EC) Directives. The MCA also supports the work of the British Pharmacopoeia Commission in setting quality standards for drug substances. The MCA is financed by fees charged to the pharmaceutical industry, but aims to set these no higher than necessary and continuously reviews the quality of its service. It is responsible for medicines control policy within the Department of Health (DH) and represents the UK in pharmaceutical regulation within European and other international settings.

During 1994, the MCA met most of its key licensing and safety targets, particularly those involving products containing new chemical entities. An MCA initiative in medical terminology (MEDDRA) has now been accepted as the basis for development of the single international medical terminology for Drug Regulatory Affairs. February saw the MCA's Medicines Inspectorate achieve international certification to International Standards Organisation (ISO) 9002, whilst in March the first ever compact disc read-only memory (CD-ROM) version of a national pharmacopoeia was issued by the British Pharmacopoeia. During the year, the Agency helped develop agreements within Europe for greater public access to information in the EC's new medicines licensing arrangements (Future Systems), whilst its European Drug Regulatory Information Service (EuroDirect) continued to be in demand.

(ii)   Control of UK clinical trials

Patients in clinical trials are protected by a system of authorisations and monitoring procedures laid down by legislation[1-4] and incorporated in guidance notes[5,6] for applicants who sponsor such trials. In 1994, the MCA approved over 270 new applications for Clinical Trial Exemptions (CTXs) and dealt with over 2,400 notifications of change to CTXs; over 4,300 adverse events and reactions were reported and assessed for drugs in clinical trials in the UK.

As part of the Government's deregulation initiative to ease the administrative burden on industry, the procedures for authorising clinical trials were reviewed. Proposals to ease the current requirements for notifying changes to clinical trials were circulated for consultation. The Guidance Notes on Applications for Clinical Trials were re-written to simplify the application procedure and to ease some requirements for pre-clinical studies. These new procedures will allow sponsors to specify limits within which changes can be made to a clinical trial without informing the Licensing Authority. Consultation on these proposals, which will not compromise the safety of patients, was completed in 1994 with a view to legislation during 1995. The European Commission announced late in 1994 that it intends to bring forward legislation to harmonise the regulation of clinical trials and standards for good clinical research practice throughout EC Member States.

(iii)   *Legal reclassification of medicinal products*

During 1994, new arrangements were introduced to publish an amendment to the Prescription Only Medicine (POM) Order[7] twice a year instead of annually, further to improve procedures for reclassification of POM medicines. This change does not affect statutory consultation requirements and evidence of safety in use remains the criterion for change. After consultation with interested organisations, the Committee on Safety of Medicines (CSM) and the Medicines Commission have released a number of medicines from prescription control. These included histamine-$_2$-receptor blockers for treating dyspepsia, substances used topically to relieve pain (piroxicam, felbinac, diclofenac), and widened indications for topical hydrocortisone to include 'mild to moderate eczema'. Nicotinic acid (when used for hyperlipidaemia) and pyrimethamine were reclassified as POM for safety reasons. The General Sales List Order was also substantially amended[8] to include a number of substances which had been temporarily approved in licensed products.

(iv)   *Pharmaceutical developments in the European Community*

The MCA maintained its leading role in the established EC licensing system during that system's final year of operation. The MCA, on behalf of the UK, was selected to be the rapporteur for nearly half of all licence applications under the old system. The other main focus of the MCA's EC work was preparation for the new EC licensing system, due to come into operation on 1 January 1995 (see page 212). The Agency negotiated Commission Regulations governing licence variations and adverse reactions reporting under the new system, and contributed to the negotiation of a Council Regulation setting fees payable to the new European Medicines Evaluation Agency (EMEA). The MCA also played an active part in the development of EC operational guidelines. It also implemented, on time, the EC legislation setting up the new system by creating a new statutory framework for the licensing and post-licensing control of most medicines in the UK, separate from the Medicines Act 1968[1] and relying on cross-reference to the relevant EC legislation.

References

1. *The Medicines Act 1968.* London: HMSO, 1968.
2. *The Medicines (Exemption from Licences) (Special Cases and Miscellaneous Provisions) Order 1972.* London: HMSO, 1972.
3. *The Medicines (Exemption from Licences)(Clinical Trials) Order 1974.* London: HMSO, 1974.
4. *The Medicines (Exemption from Licences) (Clinical Trials) Order 1981.* London: HMSO, 1981.
5. *Guidance notes on application for clinical trials certificates and clinical trial exemptions 1984.* London: HMSO, 1984.
6. *Guidance notes on applications for clinical trials certificates and clinical trial exemptions: Supplement no. 1: 1985.* London: HMSO, 1985.
7. *The Medicines (Products Other Than Veterinary Drugs) (Prescription Only) Amendment (No. 2) Order 1994.* London: HMSO, 1994 (Statutory Instrument: SI 1994 no. 3016).
8. *The Medicines (Products Other Than Veterinary Drugs) (General Sale List) Amendment Order 1994.* London: HMSO, 1994 (Statutory Instrument: SI 1994 no. 2410).

(b)   European Medicines Evaluation Agency

In 1993, the EC Council of Ministers agreed the legal framework of the EC's new medicines licensing arrangements, including the EMEA. 1994 saw much preparatory work to implement the new system before it comes into operation on 1 January 1995.

There are two new licensing procedures: a centralised procedure for certain high-technology medicines, and a decentralised procedure for other medicines. The centralised procedure will lead to the grant of a single licence valid across the EC, whereas the decentralised procedure is based on mutual recognition of national licensing decisions (with binding arbitration in the event of disagreement between Member States). The decentralised procedure will be optional until the end of 1997 for products to be marketed in more than one Member State, but national authorisation arrangements will remain for products to be marketed in just one country.

The EMEA itself acts as a secretariat, and provides administrative and technical support to these procedures - which mainly involves co-ordination of the existing scientific resources of Member States within the new procedures. In particular, EMEA supports the two committees of scientific experts nominated by the Member States to deliver opinions on licence applications and post-licensing matters; the committee that deals with medicines for use in human beings is the Committee for Proprietary Medicinal Products (CPMP).

The work during 1994 was mainly concerned with administrative preparation to establish the EMEA in London, and to ensure the new systems were ready for operation. The site for the EMEA selected by its Management Board is in Canary Wharf, London; preparation of the premises and recruitment of staff were both well advanced by the end of 1994. The EMEA will have about 130 staff initially, rising to around 200; its management board is chaired by Mr Strachan Heppell.

Setting the fees charged by the EMEA for processing applications proved difficult, and agreement was not reached in the EC Council of Ministers by the end of the year. However, no practical problems are likely to arise as these questions should be resolved early in 1995.

Although Member States will still be mainly responsible for post-licensing controls, including pharmacovigilance and inspection, the EMEA does have a role in co-ordinating work in these areas, including the development of electronic links to improve communication between Member States.

(c)   Medical Devices Agency

Next Steps Agency status

In September, the Medical Devices Directorate (MDD) became an Executive Agency of DH under the Government's 'Next Steps' initiative. The role of the Medical Devices Agency (MDA) is to safeguard the interests of patients and users of all medical devices and equipment by ensuring that such products meet appropriate standards of safety, quality and performance.

The Agency is managed by a Chief Executive, Mr Alan Kent, who is directly accountable to the Secretary of State for Health and fully responsible for the efficient management, performance and future development of the Agency. The Secretary of State for Health is assisted by an Advisory Board, chaired by Dr Jeremy Metters, Deputy Chief Medical Officer.

Developments in the EC

The UK has played an active part in bringing about a single European market in medical devices. The MDA has been involved in the negotiation and implementation of the first two of three Medical Devices Directives; the third Directive, covering in-vitro diagnostic medical devices, is still to be negotiated. The MDA acts as the UK's Competent Authority to monitor compliance with the Directives and to take any necessary enforcement action.

Active Implantable Medical Devices Directive

The transition period for this Directive finished at the end of 1994[1]; all active implantable devices subsequently on sale in the EC must carry a CE marking to show compliance with Essential Requirements for safety and performance. During 1994, two Notified Bodies were designated to authorise CE marking of active implants.

Under the provisions of this Directive, all clinical investigations of non-CE-marked devices require authorisation from the UK Competent Authority, as well as ethics committee approval. Sponsors must submit data which include a description of the device and its performance, together with a clinical investigation plan. During 1994, 12 submissions related to active implants were received, of which seven were authorised.

Medical Devices Directive

In November, Regulations to implement the provisions of the Medical Devices Directive were laid before Parliament[2], to take effect from 1 January 1995. The

MDA's principal activities with regard to this Directive were aimed at advising industry and the health service by various publications (including 17 guidance documents and bulletins); working on interpretation and resolution, such as to what extent the new Regulations would affect hospital activities; and the setting up of management systems and procedures for dealing with applications for clinical investigation, designation of Notified Bodies (6 were designated) and registration of manufacturers of Class I devices, custom-made devices and assemblers and packagers.

Adverse incident reporting centre/vigilance system

In 1994, a letter from the Chief Executive of the MDA was sent to all NHS Trust hospitals, bringing to their attention the need to report device-related adverse incidents and the systems in place for dealing with these reports.

During the year, the MDA received almost 4,000 reports of device-related adverse incidents, and investigated over 1,000 of these in depth; advice to the health service, targeted appropriately, was issued through 19 Hazard Notices and 41 Safety Action Bulletins.

With the introduction of the Medical Devices Directives, however, manufacturers will be statutorily required to report all serious incidents of CE-marked devices to the Competent Authority. Ten such reports were received in 1994.

Implants

During 1994, the MDA dealt with a number of issues related to implants. It published a comprehensive review[3] of published scientific research into silicone gel breast implants and connective tissue disease, which concluded that there was no clear evidence of a link; this report confirmed the continued validity of advice given in 1993. The MDA also issued a Safety Action Bulletin giving advice on the use of, and risks associated with, a specific type of polyurethane-coated breast implant.

During the year there was also growing concern related to the fracture of pacemaker leads. The MDA issued a Hazard Notice to draw attention to the associated risks, and to set out detailed advice on preventive measures and non-invasive diagnostic techniques for detection of any such fracture.

In addition to supporting four existing national implant registries (for heart valves, pacemakers, breast implants and hydrocephalus shunts), a new registry of neuromuscular implants was established in 1994. The information from these databases may influence policy and lead to changes in clinical practice.

Publications

During 1994, the MDA published 125 reports evaluating a wide range of devices, ranging from magnetic resonance scanners and dialysers to clinical chemistry kits and microbiology equipment. Additionally, the MDA published a booklet entitled *Doing No Harm*[4], which introduced the Agency and its functions to all professionals involved in health care.

References

1. *Active Implantable Medical Devices Regulations 1992.* London: HMSO, 1992 (Statutory Instrument: SI 1992 no. 3146).
2. *Medical Devices Regulations 1994.* London: HMSO, 1994 (Statutory Instrument: SI 1994 no. 3017).
3. Medical Devices Agency. *Evaluation of evidence for an association between implantation of silicones and connective tissue disease.* London: Department of Health, 1994.
4. Medical Devices Agency. *Doing No Harm.* London: Department of Health, 1994.

(d)   National Blood Authority

The National Blood Authority (NBA) was established in April 1993 with responsibility for the Bio-Products Laboratory (BPL), which produces blood products from donated blood, and the International Blood Group Reference Laboratory (IBGRL). From 1 April 1994, the NBA took over management responsibility for Regional Blood Transfusion Centres (RTCs) in England from Regional Health Authorities (RHAs).

The role of the NBA is to ensure that best standards are achieved uniformly through a co-ordinated National Blood Service and to enhance quality and cost effectiveness. The Authority has produced proposals to restructure the network of RTCs and is currently considering responses received during the widespread consultation on its proposals. It has appointed an independent panel to ensure that due and objective consideration is given to all comments received. The aim of these proposals is to improve the quality and service provided to hospitals, patients and blood donors; proposed changes primarily concern administration, processing and testing. The Authority has given clear assurances that hospitals will continue to receive services that are currently provided.

(e)   National Biological Standards Board

The National Biological Standards Board (NBSB) is a non-Departmental public body set up in 1976 with a statutory duty[1,2] to maintain high standards of quality and reliability of biological substances used in medicine (such as vaccines, hormones, blood products and immunological agents, which are complex entities that cannot be tested for quality by chemical analysis alone), to develop biological standards for such substances and to conduct associated research and development. The Board, which reports directly to the Secretary of State for Health, does this through its management of the National Institute for Biological Standards and Control (NIBSC).

Thus the Board and the Institute work within the Government's overall public health programme to:

-    respond to and advise on public health problems involving biological agents;

-   address new developments in science and medicine; *and*

-   take a leading role in developing the scientific basis for the control and standardisation of biological agents in Europe.

The NIBSC tests around 2,000 batches of biological substances annually - a single batch of a vaccine product can represent from 60,000 to 500,000 doses. Each year, the NIBSC prepares around 100 different standards and reference materials and distributes about 65,000 ampoules of such materials.

During 1993/94, nine NIBSC biological preparations were established by the World Health Organization (WHO) as International Standards or Reference Reagents. Major international collaborative studies leading to International Standards were completed in 1994 for inactivated poliovaccine, epidermal growth factor and human recombinant inhibin.

Between April and September, 120 batches of influenza vaccine were tested to support increased levels of vaccination in 1994/95, and the Institute completed testing of 30 batches of measles/rubella (MR) vaccine (equivalent to 15 million does of the vaccine) submitted within 15 working days of receipt of samples to support the MR vaccination campaign.

On 20 September, the NIBSC was accredited by the UK's National Measurement Accreditation Source (NAMAS) for its system of European batch release testing in 24 product areas that cover 91 separate tests and assays. The NIBSC is the first of the eight EC-designated European Control Testing Laboratories to achieve international accreditation to quality standard EN45001. The Institute has also, in collaboration with the MCA and DH, made a major input into the development of EC batch-release procedures and guidelines to manufacturers of blood products, which should make a major contribution within the EC to the viral safety of medicinal products derived from human blood and plasma. NIBSC also operated as a WHO International Laboratory for Biological Standardisation.

References

1. *Biological Standards Act 1975.* London: HMSO, 1975.
2. *National Biological Standards Board (Functions) Order 1976.* London: HMSO, 1976 (Statutory Instrument: SI 1976 no. 917).

(f)   National Radiological Protection Board

The National Radiological Protection Board (NRPB) is a non-Departmental public body which reports to the Secretary of State for Health. It is an independent statutory body set up by the Radiological Protection Act 1970[1] and the Extensions of Functions Order 1974[2].

The functions given to the Board are:

- by means of research and otherwise, to advance the acquisition of knowledge about the protection of mankind from radiation hazards (for both ionising and non-ionising radiation); *and*

- to provide information and advice to persons (including Government departments) with responsibilities in the UK in relation to the protection from radiation hazards either of the community as a whole or of particular sections of the community.

The Board was also given the power to provide technical services to persons concerned with radiation hazards and to make charges for such services and for the provision of information and advice.

The Board headquarters is in Chilton, Oxfordshire, with regional centres in Glasgow and Leeds. The principal technical services provided are radiation protection advice to a wide variety of organisations within the UK, personal dose-meters to those involved with radiation work, and radiation monitoring and instrument calibration and support.

The NRPB also contributes to the Health of the Nation initiative, particularly on skin cancer, by formal consultations, publication of advisory reports and direct provision of advice to health professionals and others involved with radiation work as well as to the general public. Training courses are also run at the NRPB and within, or in conjunction with, academic or public health institutions.

Recent formal advice includes statements on the 1990 recommendations of the International Commission on Radiological Protection[3]; on radiation exposures during pregnancy[4]; and on restrictions on human exposures to electromagnetic fields[5]. General advice has centred on occupational, public, and medical radiation exposures[6]; the health effects of visual display units[7]; and the possible risks associated with exposures to electromagnetic fields[8,9]. During 1994, guidelines were issued for the use of X-rays in primary dental care[10].

Information and advice are also made available to the general public. A range of leaflets describe topics such as medical radiation, radiation risks and non-ionising radiation. Over one million such leaflets have been produced and distributed - mainly to the public, but the leaflet on ultraviolet radiation was also sent by the Chief Medical Officer to all general practitioners in England in 1993[11] as part of DH's campaign against skin cancer.

A medical division was set up with a new medical Assistant Director from October. It is expected that this division will provide medical advice and collaborate with other divisions on projects where a medical input is required. The new medical staff will establish close links with the medical Royal Colleges and other relevant professional bodies to help practitioners keep all radiation exposures as low as reasonably practicable. It has close liaison with other Government Departments and Agencies with responsibilities in this field, such as the Health and Safety Executive for occupational exposures. The NRPB is also closely involved in the radiation monitoring programme to identify houses within radon-affected areas in the UK.

In October, Ministers thanked Sir Richard Southwood, who stood down as Chairman of the NRPB at the end of his term of office, and appointed in his place Professor Sir Keith Peters, Regius Professor of Physic, University of Cambridge, for a period of four years.

References

1. *Radiological Protection Act 1970.* London: HMSO, 1970.
2. *Extensions of Functions Order 1974.* London: HMSO, 1974.
3. National Radiological Protection Board. *Board statement on the 1990 recommendations of the International Commission on Radiological Protection.* Oxford: National Radiological Protection Board, 1993 (Doc. NRPB 4, no.1).
4. National Radiological Protection Board. *Board statement on diagnostic medical exposures to ionising radiation during pregnancy.* Oxford: National Radiological Protection Board, 1993 (Doc. NRPB 4, no. 4).
5. National Radiological Protection Board. *Board statement on restrictions on human exposure to static and time varying electromagnetic fields and radiation.* Oxford: National Radiological Protection Board, 1993 (Doc. NRPB 4, no. 5).
6. National Radiological Protection Board. *Occupational, public and medical exposure.* Oxford: National Radiological Protection Board, 1993 (Doc. NRPB 4, no. 2).
7. National Radiological Protection Board. *Health effects related to the use of visual display units: report of an advisory group on non-ionising radiation.* Oxford: National Radiological Protection Board, 1994 (Doc. NRPB 5, no. 2).
8. National Radiological Protection Board. *Electromagnetic fields and the risk of cancer: report of the Advisory Group on Non-ionising Radiation.* Oxford: National Radiological Protection Board, 1994 (Doc. NRPB 5, no. 2). Chair: Sir Richard Doll.
9. National Radiological Protection Board. *Electromagnetic fields and the risk of cancer: supplementary report by the Advisory Group on Non-ionising Radiation.* Oxford: National Radiological Protection Board, 1994 (Doc. NRPB 5, no. 2).
10. Royal College of Radiologists, National Radiological Protection Board. *Guidelines of radiology standards for primary dental care.* Oxford: National Radiological Protection Board, 1994 (Doc. NRPB 5, no. 3).
11. Department of Health. *Ultraviolet radiation and skin cancer.* Heywood (Lancashire): Department of Health, 1993 (Professional Letter: PL/CMO(93)6).

(g)   United Kingdom Transplant Support Service Authority

The UK Transplant Support Service Authority (UKTSSA) was established as a Special Health Authority on 1 April 1991 to provide a 24-hour support service to all transplant units in the UK and Republic of Ireland, taking over the work of the UK Transplant Service. Its main functions include the matching and allocation of organs for transplantation on an equitable basis and in accordance with agreed methodologies; the provision of support and quality assurance to local tissue-typing laboratories; the maintenance and analysis of the national database of transplant information; and the production of audit reports on the status of transplantation and organ donation and use. The UKTSSA also provides a forum at which transplant and organ donation issues can be discussed and is responsible for the maintenance of the National Health Service (NHS) Organ Donor Register, which was established in 1994. During the year the authority was awarded the Crown Emblem.

(h)   Microbiological Research Authority

After a Government review, the Centre for Applied Microbiology and Research (CAMR) was transferred out of the Public Health Laboratory Service (PHLS) and made a Special Health Authority in its own right from 1 April. The Board of this new Microbiological Research Authority (MRA) was appointed by, and reports to, DH Ministers.

Since its creation as a Ministry of Defence establishment in 1951, CAMR had built up an international reputation through the development of vaccines and therapeutic and diagnostic agents. Whilst continuing to develop its expertise in the pathogenesis and diagnosis of infectious disease in human beings, the MRA is increasingly able to apply the results of this work for use by the biopharmaceuticals industry. Public health research at MRA includes major projects related to HIV, *Salmonella, Campylobacter*, verocytotoxin-producing *Escherichia coli* (VTEC) and *Legionella* infections. An important venture for 1995 will be involvement in a new DH initiative to evaluate combination vaccines for use in children.

(i)   Creutzfeldt-Jakob Disease Surveillance Unit

The Creutzfeldt-Jakob Disease (CJD) Surveillance Unit was established in Edinburgh in 1990 to monitor any changes in the pattern of CJD in the UK, after a recommendation by the Working Party on Bovine Spongiform Encephalopathy (BSE), set up in 1988 to examine the implications of BSE for human and animal health. The Unit is funded jointly by the DH and the Scottish Office Home and Health Department.

Suspected and definite cases of CJD, including iatrogenic and familial cases, are reported to the Unit by clinicians throughout the UK (see Table 9.1): these cases undergo detailed clinical and neuropathological investigation with particular attention paid to the study of putative risk factors, including dietary and occupational history. No conclusive evidence of any change in CJD that could be attributable to BSE has yet been found, but surveillance will need to continue for some years in view of the potentially prolonged incubation period of CJD.

(j)   Bioethics

(i)   *Local Research Ethics Committees*

DH guidelines issued in 1991 required each District Health Authority (DHA) to establish a Local Research Ethics Committee (LREC). In 1994, DH issued a Standards Framework[1] for ethical review and material on standard operating procedures to promote good and nationally consistent practice by LRECs; these were publicised in regional workshops. The documents set out the objectives of LRECs and can be used to identify training needs and scope for improvement through managerial action[2].

Table 9.1: *Creutzfeldt-Jakob disease (CJD) and Gerstmann-Straussler-Scheinker syndrome (GSS), United Kingdom, 1985-94*

Year	Creutzfeldt-Jakob disease			GSS	Total	Sporadic incidence/ million population*
	Sporadic	Iatrogenic	Familial			
1985	26	1	1	0	28	0.45
1986	26	0	0	0	26	0.45
1987	23	0	0	1	24	0.40
1988	21	1	1	0	23	0.36
1989	28	1	1	0	30	0.48
1990	26	5	0	0	31	0.45
1991	32	1	3	0	36	0.55
1992	44	2	4	1	51	0.76
1993	35	4	2	1	42	0.61
1994	53	1	0	1	55	0.92

*Based on UK population of 57.78 million (1991 Census Update).

Note: These figures may differ from those published previously because the Unit is still identifying cases from previous years.

Source: UK CJD Surveillance Unit

The Chief Medical Officer convened a consultative group to consider options for change in November, building on previous consultation on training for LRECs; methods to streamline procedures to ease the process of ethical approval for multi-centre research span a large number of DHAs.

(ii) Bioethics in Europe

The Council of Europe's Steering Committee on Bioethics (CDBI) is charged by the Council of Ministers to study the impact of progress in biomedical sciences on law, ethics, and human rights. The working party of CDBI chaired by Dr Michael Abrams (formerly Deputy Chief Medical Officer) continued to develop a framework Bioethics Convention; a draft was issued for consultation in July. Three protocols - on organ transplantation, medical research, and the protection of the human embryo and the foetus - are planned under the Convention, which emphasises the need to protect those who lack capacity to give consent.

(iii) Genetic screening

Last year's Report[3] recorded increasing interest in the ethical issues raised by genetic screening, and noted the publication of the Nuffield Council on Bioethics Report, *Genetic Screening: ethical issues*[4]. During 1994, DH had informal discussions with representatives of other Government Departments, the Association of British Insurers (ABI) and medical professional bodies.

The House of Commons Select Committee on Science and Technology began its Inquiry into Human Genetics - a wide-ranging Inquiry which will encompass genetic screening. The report of the Committee, due in 1995, will inform and stimulate the wider Parliamentary and public discussion of the ethical issues.

(iv) Draft guidance on confidentiality

In August, DH issued draft guidance on the confidentiality, use and disclosure of personal health information for wide consultation. The purpose of the draft guidance is to ensure that, in the interests of patients, personal health information is handled confidentially and in accordance with strict safeguards. The guidance is based on the common law duty of confidence, and takes careful account of the ethical obligations of health professionals.

A key element is the need to ensure that information is made available to patients about the uses of personal health information, and about the organisations to which it might be disclosed. The draft guidance emphasises that personal information may be disclosed within the NHS only on a strict need-to-know basis, and must be anonymised unless the recipient has to know the patient's identity. Patient information may not be disclosed outside the NHS unless the patient consents, or unless disclosure is required by Statute or Court Order, or can be justified in the public interest.

The Department received over 170 responses to the consultation, which reflected the sensitivity of this complex legal and ethical issue. The responses are being analysed and it is intended that definitive guidance will be issued during 1995.

(v) House of Lords Select Committee on Medical Ethics

After an extensive examination of issues concerning the end of life, the House of Lords Select Committee on Medical Ethics reported in January[5]. The Committee recommended no change to the law on euthanasia and on assisted suicide, and rejected calls for an offence of 'mercy killing'. The Government response strongly supported the Committee's view[6].

The Committee commended the development of advance directives which would enable people to express views on their health care should they lose decision-making capacity in the future. Following the Committee's recommendation, the British Medical Association (BMA) set up a working group (with a DH observer) to develop a code of practice on advance directives.

The Committee also recommended the development of a code of practice on the persistent vegetative state; this work was subsequently taken forward by the Royal College of Physicians of London.

References

1. Department of Health. *Standards for Local Research Ethics Committees: a framework for ethical review*. London: Department of Health, 1994.
2. Bendall C. *Standard operating procedures for Local Research Ethics Committees*. London: McKenna, 1994.
3. Department of Health. *On the State of the Public Health: the annual report of the Chief Medical Officer of the Department of Health for the year 1993*. London: HMSO, 1994; 135-6.
4. Nuffield Council on Bioethics. *Genetic screening: ethical issues: report of a working party*. London: Nuffield Council on Bioethics, 1993. Chair: Professor Dame June Lloyd.
5. House of Lords. Select Committee on Medical Ethics. *Report of the Select Committee on Medical Ethics: Volume 1: 1994*. London: HMSO, 1994. Chair: Baron Walton of Detchant.
6. Department of Health. *Government response to the report of the Select Committee on Medical Ethics*. London: HMSO, 1994 (Cm. 2553).

(k) Research and development

(i) White Paper on Science, Engineering and Technology

The 1993 White Paper *Realising Our Potential: a strategy for science, engineering and technology*[1] was the first major Governmental policy review of science and technology for over 20 years, and aimed to help the scientific, engineering and business communities to secure the maximum economic benefit from science and technology, whilst continuing to support excellence in basic research. Stronger links between industrial and Government science and technology strategy were highlighted, and the contribution of advances in health technologies to the wealth-creating capacity of the nation through improved services and quality of life were noted.

The White Paper's strategic approach was mirrored in the development of the Department's own research and development (R&D) strategy. The publication of the first *Forward Look of Government funded science, engineering and technology* in April[2] provided an opportunity to consider future R&D challenges for the Department in health and medicine. The second Forward Look, due to be published in May 1995, will be strengthened by the results of the Technology Foresight Programme (TFP), which seeks to identify scientific and technological areas of opportunity which will contribute to future wealth creation and improvements in the quality of life. Health and life sciences is the subject of a separate TFP panel, which has reviewed long-term trends and assessed principal opportunities and challenges and is due to report in Spring 1995.

The new Council for Science and Technology (CST) established by the White Paper[1] aims to ensure that the Government benefits from outside independent and expert advice when deciding on its own research spending priorities. It includes members from the health and medical field and has taken a keen interest in health research.

(ii)   Research for health

Research for health[3], published in June 1993, set the direction for DH's R&D strategy, including the wider R&D Strategy, research in the NHS, and the Department's Centrally Commissioned Programme (CCP). The overall strategy is designed to provide a coherent, research-led approach to the challenges that DH and the NHS will face in the 21st century.

DH's centrally commissioned research programme policy provides knowledge for evidence-based development of health service policy, social services policy and central policy directed at the health and well-being of the whole population. To enhance its impact, research is focused on a range of strategic programmes that cover Ministers' central responsibilities. Priority criteria are: relevance to these central responsibilities; the actual or potential burden of a problem; timeliness; research feasibility; return on investment; and appropriateness for DH priority. Future programmes of work now in the planning stage will focus on child care, community health services, prescribing and vaccine development.

(iii)   Developments in the NHS research and development programme

The aim of the NHS R&D strategy is to secure a knowledge-based health service in which clinical, managerial and policy decisions are based on sound and relevant information about research findings and scientific developments as set out in *Research for health*[3]. The proposed changes in the structure of the NHS, and the report of the NHS R&D Task Force, have provided opportunities to improve the management of the programme. The document *Research and development in the new NHS*[4] describes how R&D will be organised within the new framework.

Following publication in December of *Supporting research and development in the NHS*[5], the report of the NHS R&D Task Force, chaired by Professor Anthony Culyer, the Secretary of State for Health announced a radical new 'single stream' funding mechanism for NHS R&D, with funds raised by a levy on purchasers of health care from 1996/97 and distributed through contracts to support work initiated by the NHS and by other funders.

The Central Research and Development Committee (CRDC) continues to advise on priorities for centrally funded research. In 1994, new centrally funded NHS research programmes have been established in physical and complex disabilities, the primary/secondary care interface, health technology assessment and cancer.

The NHS R&D Information Systems Strategy continues to bring information about R&D findings to the attention of decision-makers in the NHS. Within this strategy, the UK Cochrane Centre and the NHS Centre for Reviews and Dissemination have made considerable progress in developing their role to provide, maintain and disseminate systematic reviews of reliable evidence from around the world about the effects of individual health care interventions.

References

1. Office of Public Service and Science. *Realising Our Potential: a strategy for science, engineering and technology.* London: HMSO, 1993 (Cm. 2250).
2. Cabinet Office, Office of Public Service and Science, Office of Science and Technology. *Forward Look of Government funded science, engineering and technology.* London: HMSO, 1994.
3. Department of Health. *Research for health.* London: Department of Health, 1993.
4. NHS Management Executive. *Research and development in the new NHS: functions and responsibilities.* Leeds: Department of Health, 1994.
5. Research and Development Task Force. *Supporting research and development in the NHS.* London: HMSO, 1994. Chair: Professor Anthony Culyer.

(l)   Dental health

(i)   *Dental health of the nation*

An oral health strategy for England[1] was published alongside the Green Paper *Improving NHS Dentistry*[2]. The strategy reviews the present state of oral health in England, highlights problem areas, indicates in broad terms how these might be tackled and sets national objectives for future improvements in oral health. It states that future emphasis should be on the early detection and prevention of oral diseases, viewed in the context of the health of individuals as a whole, and on quality of care rather than quantity.

In December, the third in a series of decennial surveys of children's dental health was published by the Office of Population Censuses and Surveys (OPCS)[3]. The survey showed increasing numbers of caries-free children throughout the country. Encouraging findings included:

-       the proportion of 5-year-old children in England estimated to have at least one decayed deciduous tooth had fallen from 48% to 44%;

- active decay in permanent teeth had decreased for all groups with the greatest fall among older children. English children had the lowest prevalence of active tooth decay: for example, at the age of 8 years 11% of children in England had active decay, compared with 19% of children in Northern Ireland;

- the proportion of children with filled permanent teeth significantly decreased in every age group; from the age of 8 years upwards, children in England had the lowest proportion of filled teeth. At 10 years-of-age just 16% of children had one or more permanent teeth filled in 1993, compared with 45% in 1983; among 15-year-olds the reduction was from 85% to 45%; *and*

- extractions of permanent teeth due to decay had become less frequent among children of every age-group from 8 years upwards. Only 1 in 20 of 15-year-olds had lost teeth due to decay in 1993, compared with 21% in 1983.

However, some findings were more disappointing:

- there was no change in the total tooth decay experience of 5-year-olds since 1983;

- 70% of dental caries among 5-year-olds was untreated;

- 28% of dental caries among 15-year-olds was untreated;

- there had been virtually no change in the periodontal condition of 15-year-olds since 1983 (in 1993, 8% showed evidence of gingivitis and periodontal pocketing, compared with 7% in 1983);

- 15% of 15-year-olds needed orthodontic treatment;

- the level of dental erosion due to acidic carbonated drinks was a cause for concern; *and*

- only 31% of incisors damaged by trauma had been treated.

The results of the survey indicate more than ever that a need remains for population-based preventive measures, such as water fluoridation, effective oral health education and an improved capitation payment system for treating children.

(ii)   General dental services

The Green Paper *Improving NHS Dentistry*[2], published on 14 July in response to Sir Kenneth Bloomfield's fundamental review of dental remuneration[4], set out the Government's proposals for reform of the dental remuneration system. The proposals are intended to implement the Government's commitment to an effective and accessible NHS dental service for all those who need it, and underline the importance of a continuing improvement in the oral health of children. The Government's overall objective in proposing reform is to create a system of remuneration which provides value for money within a proper framework of financial control; is fair to dentists, patients and the taxpayer; is as simple as possible; and contributes positively to the development of the NHS dental service and oral health generally. The proposals also draw heavily on the recommendations of the 1993 Report of the Health Select Committee[5,6].

For the long term, the Green Paper proposes that NHS dental care could be provided through a system of local purchasing by health authorities. In principle, the benefits of identifying priorities and quality standards to be achieved and then encapsulating these in contracts should increase the health gain to be derived from the resources available. Subject to Parliamentary approval, this approach would be piloted over two years and then be subject to rigorous evaluation before deciding whether and how to implement such a system nationwide. Two further options are proposed for improving the system while this long-term option is being developed: a sessional fee model would reward dentists for the time spent with NHS patients rather than the number of treatments performed; another option would be to modify the present fee-per-item system of remuneration.

The publication of the Green Paper was followed by a period of formal consultation which invited the views of all interested parties. The consultation ended on 1 November and the Government is now considering the result.

Gross expenditure on general dental services in 1993/94, although lower than the previous year when payments to dentists exceeded expected amounts, was still 24% higher in real terms than in 1983/84. The proportion of gross costs met from charges to patients increased from 27% to 30% over the decade, but has fallen from a peak 39% in 1989/90, largely due to the introduction in 1990 of continuing care payments for registered adults (for which there is no patient charge).

(iii)   Community dental services

The provision of community dental services (CDS) is now firmly established within NHS Trusts providing services to local populations. The service continues to develop but retains responsibility for monitoring the dental health of the population; the provision of dental health education and preventive programmes; the provision of treatment for special categories of patients; and the screening of children's teeth in state-funded schools. Purchasing of dental services to meet local need is carried out on the advice of consultants in dental public health and, in some cases, chief administrative dental officers and district dental officers. Purchasers seeking improvements in the quality of services they obtain may invite bids for particular services.

The total number of community dental staff in Great Britain fell from 1,820 to 1,780 in the year to 30 September 1993. The delivery of community dental services is usually managed by a district dental officer, service director or manager who may also carry out clinical work. The bulk of clinical work is undertaken by both senior dental officers and community dental officers.

Within the Green Paper *Improving NHS Dentistry*[2], the Government recognised the importance of the 'safety-net' function of the community dental services and salaried dentists employed by Family Health Services Authorities (FHSAs), but considered that it made little sense for there to be two quite separate groups of dentists providing that safety net. In those parts of the country where, at any given time, the general dental services (GDS) provision is not fully adequate for all who wish to make use of it, the role of the CDS would be strengthened. Additionally, the Government would propose amending legislation to allow the CDS to levy charges similar to those applicable in the GDS on patients not otherwise exempt.

(iv)   Hospital dental services

The number of hospital dentists in England rose by 2.6% from 1,238 whole-time equivalent posts to 1,270 between September 1992 and September 1993. There were 422 consultants in post, a decrease of 4.7% over the previous year. The number of senior registrars rose from 98 to 112, and the number of senior house officers rose by 17.1% from 251 to 294.

Compared with 1992/93, there was a fall in new outpatient referrals to consultant clinics of 1.1% in 1993/94. In oral surgery, referrals rose by 1.5% from 394,268 to 400,123, and in orthodontics referrals rose by 2% from 103,625 to 105,709. In restorative dentistry, referrals fell by 18.5% from 59,074 to 48,126 and referrals in paediatric dentistry fell by 12.6% from 27,685 to 24,193. Over the same time, repeat attendances at outpatient clinics rose by 0.6%. Repeat attendances rose by 1.5% in orthodontics from 657,968 to 667,859, and by 3.7% in restorative dentistry from 339,363 to 352,003. Repeat attendances fell by 0.9% from 727,773 to 721,494 in oral surgery, and by 6.5% from 79,358 to 74,237 in paediatric dentistry.

(v)   Continuing education and training for dentists

There were 513 trainees in 47 regionally based vocational training schemes on 1 October.

The Committee for Continuing Education and Training identified the following priority areas for the training of general dental practitioners in 1994/95: supporting the oral health strategy; the Nutrition Task Force's curriculum for health care professionals; 'hands-on' courses; the management of elderly or disabled patients and those with special needs; sedation techniques, pain control and the management of anxious patients; courses to reinforce distance learning programmes; the training of trainers, advisers and examiners; research techniques relevant to general dental practice; training practice support staff; and courses which promote peer review and clinical audit in general dental practice. These courses are arranged by regional postgraduate dental deans or directors of dental education and funded by DH under the provisions of Section 63 of the Health Services and Public Health Act 1968[7].

During 1994, DH continued to fund the production and distribution of distance learning material to general dental practices, including four computer assisted learning programmes: 'Aspects of partial denture design', 'Minimal preparation resin retained bridgework', 'Molar endodontics' and 'The management of patients with special needs'.

(vi)   Dental research

Diet and the oral health of people aged 65 years and over

A team from University College London, Social and Community Planning and Research (SCPR) and the Universities of Newcastle-upon-Tyne and Birmingham was commissioned to conduct a national survey on the condition and function of the tissues in the mouths of a sample of subjects aged 65 years or over. During 1995, approximately 1,100 individuals, selected at random in England, Scotland and Wales, will be examined in four equal groups at three-monthly intervals. The survey is to be carried out in the subject's home or long-stay institution and consists of a dental examination together with an interview based on a dental and dietary questionnaire. Data from this survey will be correlated with information gathered from a more detailed nutritional survey of the same sample group as part of the National Diet and Nutritional Survey Programme.

Dental crowns

The report[8] of a follow-up to the 1988 Adult Dental Health Survey[9], conducted by the Social Survey Division of OPCS on behalf of DH, was published in November. This dealt with the findings among almost 600 people in England who had at some time had a tooth crowned and asked them to recall the history of their crowned teeth. More than half the sample surveyed reported having crowns which had lasted at least 15 years.

References

1. Department of Health. *An oral health strategy for England.* London: Department of Health, 1994.
2. Department of Health. *Improving NHS Dentistry.* London: HMSO, 1994 (Cm. 2625).
3. O'Brien M. *Children's dental health in the United Kingdom 1993: a survey carried out by the Social Survey Division of OPCS, on behalf of the United Kingdom health departments, in collaboration with the dental schools at the Universities of Birmingham and Newcastle.* London: HMSO, 1994.
4. Department of Health. *Fundamental Review of Dental Remuneration: report of Sir Kenneth Bloomfield KCB.* London: Department of Health, 1992.
5. House of Commons. Health Committee. *Dental Services: fourth report from the Health Committee: Session 1992-93.* London: HMSO, 1993. Chair: Ms Marion Roe. (HC 264, vols I-II).
6. Department of Health. *Government Response to the fourth report from the Health Committee: Session 1992-93: dental services.* London: HMSO, 1993 (Cm. 2308).
7. *Health Services and Public Health Act 1968.* London: HMSO, 1968.
8. Todd J, Lader D, Dodd T. *Dental crowns: report of a follow-up to the 1988 adult health survey.* London: HMSO, 1994.
9. Todd J, Lader D. *Adult dental health: United Kingdom 1988.* London: HMSO, 1991.

CHAPTER 10

INTERNATIONAL HEALTH

(a)   England, Europe and health

Many of the health challenges encountered in England and the United Kingdom (UK) as a whole are also found in the rest of Europe. Diseases have little respect for national boundaries. The pace of technological advance, ageing populations and rising expectations lead to growing demands on health care services throughout Europe and beyond. The challenge of drug dependence is also a shared one.

The opportunity to work together on common problems within the European Community (EC), and in international bodies such as the World Health Organization (WHO) and the Council of Europe, brings great benefits. The UK has much expertise to offer on health matters, but can also benefit greatly from the knowledge of others, from the insight of international comparisons, and from the greater resources that international co-operation can bring into play.

Nowhere can be insulated from the changes taking place in the world. Political change in central and eastern Europe opens up the prospect of much greater freedom of movement including trade relations, but has also produced dislocation in which old diseases have re-emerged and health care has deteriorated. Migration to the EC has grown rapidly, bringing groups who have distinct health needs and present new challenges to the public health systems of host countries.

(b)   The European Community

(i)   *The Council of Health Ministers*

The Council of Ministers is a key decision-making body of the EC, in which all Member States are represented. Councils of Ministers with particular responsibilities, such as health, meet regularly to deal with relevant EC business.

In 1994, the Health Council held general meetings on 2 June and 22 December. These took forward proposals for EC action in line with the Framework Action in the Field of Public Health published in November 1993[1]. By the end of the year, four areas were being explored: extension of the 'Europe against Cancer' programme, and work on AIDS and other communicable diseases, on drug dependence and on health promotion. The cancer proposals are closest to adoption and should be implemented during 1995.

The Health Council also held special meetings to exchange information on bovine spongiform encephalopathy (BSE) and on precautions to be taken following the outbreak of bubonic plague in India.

(ii)   EC/WHO/Council of Europe

Close co-operation between the EC, the WHO and the Council of Europe continued during 1994. Examples of collaboration included joint EC/WHO sponsorship of the Conference on Environment and Health in Helsinki (see page 194), and the development for the EC by WHO's Regional Office for Europe of pilot projects for information networks in communicable diseases, health statistics, pharmacovigilance and other health-related areas. The EC also worked closely with the Council of Europe to promote European self-sufficiency in blood and blood products.

Once again, assistance to Central and Eastern Europe was a major field of collaboration involving WHO's EUROHEALTH programme for this region and the EC's PHARE (Poland and Hungary Assistance for Economic Restructuring, which despite the name now operates throughout central Europe) and TACIS (Technical Assistance to the Commonwealth of Independent States) programmes.

(iii)   European Economic Area

The European Economic Area (EEA), which came into being on 1 January 1994, extended the Single European Market to Austria, Finland, Iceland, Norway and Sweden. Virtually all the EC's rules on free movement of goods, services, people and capital now apply throughout this area. Provisions related to health include the mutual recognition of professional qualifications, and the regulation of food safety and pharmaceuticals.

For Austria, Finland and Sweden, membership of the EEA was a staging post on the way to full EC membership, which will be achieved on 1 January 1995. For Norway, which voted in a referendum not to join the EC, and for Iceland, the EEA continues to provide closer ties with EC countries than ever before. Liechtenstein is likely to join the EEA during 1995.

(iv)   Free movement of people

Health professionals

The number of health professionals from other EEA Member States working in the UK is small and most come for short periods to gain experience. In 1994, 1,471 doctors with qualifications from other Member States obtained full registration with the General Medical Council, 129 dentists with the General Dental Council, 22 pharmacists with the Royal Pharmaceutical Society of Great Britain, 437 nurses and 19 midwives with the UK Central Council of Nursing, Midwifery and Health Visiting, and 449 persons with the Council for the Professions Supplementary to Medicine (comprising 3 chiropodists, 64 occupational therapists, 29 dietitians, 342 physiotherapists and 11 radiographers).

Patients

EC Social Security Regulation 1408/71 continued to operate satisfactorily, co-ordinating health care cover for people moving between EEA Member States. The main categories covered were temporary visitors, detached workers and pensioners transferring their residence to another Member State. In 1994, 580 applications by UK patients for referral to other Member States specifically for treatment of pre-existing conditions were approved by DH. About 310 citizens of other Member States were treated in the UK on the same basis.

(v) Channel Tunnel and port health checks

The Channel Tunnel opened for business in 1994, thereby establishing for the first time a physical link between the UK and continental Europe, including the use of international trains.

The Public Health (International Trains) Regulations 1994[2,3] provide for the protection of public health in the UK by requiring operators of the Channel Tunnel and international rail service to take appropriate remedial action in the unlikely event of an incident - for example the sighting of a rodent or small animal, or the suspicion of a passenger with a serious communicable disease on any of the trains. These measures do not put any unnecessary burden on the operators, or on the responsible enforcing authorities. Health control units set up at Waterloo International Terminal in London, Cheriton in Kent and Coquelles, near Calais, France comply with the statutory responsibility of the Secretary of State for Health under the Immigration Act 1971[4] to provide for the medical inspection of entrants into the UK.

(vi) Draft Directive on Data Protection

Negotiations on the Directive continued during 1994. The Directive seeks to establish a common set of rules for the protection of personal data held on computer or in manual records. The intention is to ensure that an equivalent level of protection exists in all Member States, to facilitate the transfer of such personal data across national boundaries within the EC. As originally drafted, the Directive was very prescriptive and bureaucratic, and the Government was concerned at the costs, administrative burdens, and possible barriers to medical research that the Directive would place on public and private sectors alike. The text has been considerably changed in the course of negotiations, and helpful amendments with regard to health data were agreed during 1994.

(vii) Smoking

Several aspects of EC activity are relevant to tobacco consumption in individual Member States. Price is a particularly powerful determinant of tobacco consumption, and EC rules on excise duties are important. These do not at present provide sufficient upward pressure on tobacco prices, but negotiations to review the excise rules were postponed to 1995. The new EC programme of actions against cancer included proposals to exchange information about measures to reduce tobacco consumption. The Health Council also held a further discussion of the Commission's proposal to ban tobacco advertising. The UK and others continue to oppose the measure on the grounds that this is an area where EC countries should be free to decide what controls are likely to be most effective in the light of national circumstances. The Commission will now consider how to move forward.

(viii)   Elderly and disabled people

An evaluation of the 1993 'European Year of Older People and Solidarity Between Generations' was undertaken in the UK and across the EC. The year was the culmination of a three-year programme of measures to encourage the transfer of knowledge, ideas and experience about ageing between Member States. The evaluation report considered "the overwhelming response from the grassroots to the initiative is in itself an indication of success". To mark the end of the programme a Declaration of Principles, signed by all Member States, was produced and the Commission has drawn up proposals for a second programme of Community actions in this area.

The third EC Action Programme to assist disabled people, HELIOS II, involved some 78 UK organisations in study visits to other Member States to consider examples of good practice in the areas of social and educational integration and functional and employment rehabilitation.

(ix)   AIDS and HIV infection

Support continued during 1994 for actions under the 'Europe Against AIDS' programme, which was extended to the end of 1995 by a Health Council decision in December, allowing the EC to continue these actions until a new programme, covering not only AIDS but a range of other communicable diseases, is adopted.

On World AIDS Day, held on 1 December, the Secretary of State for Health represented the UK at a meeting called by France to consider strategies for future co-operation against AIDS world wide.

(x)   Research and information technology

EC research and development is encompassed within medium-term Framework Programmes: the Fourth Framework Programme (FP4) covering 1994-98 has now been agreed and new research proposals will be considered shortly. Three areas in FP4 are of particular interest to DH: Biomedicine and Health (BIOMED), Telematics (through initiatives in health care informatics and systems to assist disabled and elderly people), and the Nuclear Fission Safety Programme. BIOMED aims to respond to the challenges that rapidly emerging health technologies and new epidemics pose in Europe: the needs of patients, health care professionals, health industries and the EC as a whole will be emphasised.

(xi) *Food safety*

The EC General Food Hygiene Directive, adopted in June 1993, set out general hygiene principles and conditions for foodstuffs. Draft Food Safety (General Food Hygiene) Regulations, which implement this Directive, were issued for information in September 1994, and set out the general hygiene principles and conditions for foodstuffs to apply throughout the food chain after harvesting or slaughter. They are scheduled to come into force in September 1995.

A number of industry sectors are developing voluntary guides to good practice, a feature of the Regulations, which are intended to provide guidance on compliance with the new Regulations - particularly the new requirements for staff hygiene training and the need for food businesses to identify and to control critical food safety steps.

With the implementation of this Directive, nearly all food hygiene Directives will have been implemented into UK law by the end of 1995.

Directive on Scientific Co-operation in the Examination of Questions Relating to Food

This Directive allows scientific bodies nominated by Member States to carry out food safety evaluations on behalf of the EC. The UK is co-ordinating a task on food temperature control, for completion in September 1995.

(xii) *Medical Devices Directives*

The transitional period of the Active Implantable Medical Devices Directive (90/385/EEC) expired on 31 December; all such devices must carry the CE marking from 1 January 1995.

The Medical Devices Directive (93/42/EEC) comes into effect on 1 January 1995 and will have a transitional period to 13 June 1998, during which time manufacturers may choose to follow either existing national rules in force or the provisions of the Directive. The Medical Devices Regulations 1994 (SI 94/3017) which will implement the provisions of this Directive in the UK were laid before Parliament on 30 November (see page 213).

References

1. Commission of the European Communities. *Commission communication on the framework for action in the field of public health.* Luxembourg: Office for Official Publications of the EC, 1993 (COM(93); 559 final).
2. *The Public Health (International Trains) Regulations 1994.* London: HMSO, 1994 (Statutory Instrument: SI 1994 no. 311).
3. *The Public Health (International Trains) Regulations 1994 (as amended by Statutory Instrument: SI 1994/1405).* London: HMSO, 1994 (Statutory Instrument: SI 1994 no. 1405).
4. Immigration Act 1971. London: HMSO, 1971.

(c)   Relations with Central and Eastern Europe

A visit to Kazakhstan by representatives of DH, the Overseas Development Administration (ODA) and the World Bank took place in February, and resulted in a paper on proposed strategy and health sector issues. The first phase of the implementation of this strategy was launched in the form of a workshop in Almaty in November. A number of follow-up projects have already been set up, covering issues such as management training for chief doctors. In March, the Secretary of State for Health met President Nazarbaev of Kazakhstan in Downing Street; DH also hosted a visit from the Health Minister of Kyrgyzstan, Mr Naken Kasiev.

There continue to be active Health Co-operation Agreements with Bulgaria, the Czech and Slovak Republics, Hungary, Poland, Romania, and Russia. A Plan of Co-operation under the new Agreement with Russia was signed at the May World Health Assembly in Geneva. During the year, revised Plans were also signed with Poland and Hungary.

Exchanges with Central and Eastern European countries included visits to the UK to attend courses and conferences. Specialists from Bulgaria, the Czech Republic, Romania and Russia took part, with topics including services for people with multiple disabilities, psychiatry, nursing and the delivery of health care. From Hungary, the UK received visitors interested in general practice and health visiting; paediatric neonatology was a topic favoured by the Poles; projects related to cystic fibrosis and paediatric nursing attracted visits from Russia; and the Slovak Republic explored specialist expertise in hepatobiliary surgery.

UK specialists visited Central and Eastern Europe to advise and exchange information on various topics. Health service management, health education, and the genetics of manic depressive illness were covered in Bulgaria; in the Czech Republic, a summer school on epidemiology and public health was organised; neonatology, gastroenterology, health education and cystic fibrosis were among topics covered by visitors to Poland; and psychopathology and psychology were the main areas of interest for visitors to Romania. Academic links in orthopaedics were established between Aberdeen and Bucharest. Projects agreed with the Russians covered cystic fibrosis, nursing and infection control.

During 1994, the EC concluded 'Europe Agreements' with Bulgaria, the Czech Republic, Hungary, Poland, Romania and Slovakia. These go further than previous agreements by acknowledging an ultimate goal of eligibility for membership of the European Union. To this end, these six countries will work towards making their administrative and legal systems compatible with all areas of EC law, and receive assistance to do so. They are also free to participate in EC programmes, including those now being negotiated in public health. Funds from the PHARE programme are available to assist in the costs of this process.

(d)   Council of Europe

The Steering Committee on Bioethics (CDBI) studied the impact of progress in biomedical sciences and law, ethics and human rights (see page 221). The working party of CBDI, chaired by Dr Michael Abrams (formerly Deputy Chief Medical Officer), continued to develop a framework Bioethics Convention; a draft was issued for consultation in July. Three protocols - on organ transplantation, medical research and the protection of the human embryo and the foetus - are planned under the Convention, which emphasises the need to protect those who lack capacity to give consent.

Work was taken forward in developing a draft Recommendation aimed at safeguarding medical data. In common with the Data Protection Act in the UK, the Recommendation will apply to computerised health data, though Member States may apply it to paper records if they choose. The draft Recommendation contains principles on the circumstances in which health data may be processed or communicated, and the rights of the individual to have access to his or her data.

Another key area of work has been the progressive development of the European Pharmacopoeia. During 1994, the European Union acceded to the convention on the elaboration of a European Pharmacopoeia; and the number of Member States increased to 23 with the accession of Croatia, Turkey and the former Yugoslav Republic of Macedonia. Australia, Canada and China were granted observer status. Monographs in the 17th Fascicule of the second edition of the European Pharmacopoeia were implemented on 1 January, and notice was given that monographs and other texts published during 1994 in the 18th Fascicule would be implemented from 1 January 1995.

The Council of Europe Pompidou Group held its 10th Ministerial Conference and 2nd Pan-European Ministerial Conference in February. Mr John Bowis MP, Parliamentary Under Secretary of State for Health in the House of Commons, represented the UK. He welcomed the Group's proposed Work Programme for 1994-97, which gives a greater emphasis to work to prevent drug misuse as well as to control supply. DH is involved in several of the Pompidou working groups including those on epidemiology, treatment and rehabilitation, new developments in drug misuse, and training.

The UK contributed to and supported the Council of Europe in their work on blood, blood safety, organ transplantation and xenotransplantation.

(e)   Organization for Economic Co-operation and Development

The Organization for Economic Co-operation and Development (OECD), which brings together nearly all European countries and the other large industrialised countries of the world, has developed in recent years a valuable expertise in health reform and the financing of health care. In November, the OECD held a conference of national experts on healthcare reform in Paris. The Secretary of

State for Health led the UK delegation and described British experiences of health system reform. Issues discussed at this conference and in OECD's publications on health matters during the year included evidence-based care, medical technology, rationing, the funding of long-term care, and the safeguarding of quality of care during times of cost restraint.

(f)   The Commonwealth

Commonwealth Health Ministers met in Geneva on 1 May, before the World Health Assembly. The UK delegation was led by the Chief Medical Officer and included the Chief Nursing Officer and a representative from the Health and Population Division of the Overseas Development Administration. The Chief Medical Officer gave a report on progress and the recommendations of the Working Group he chaired on WHO's response to global change. Other issues discussed covered maternal and child health, including mid-decade goals for child survival and issues related to AIDS. Observer status was granted to the Commonwealth Dental Association and the United Nations International Children's Emergency Fund (UNICEF); South Africa also attended in this capacity pending its return to the Commonwealth on 1 June.

(g)   World Health Organization

(i)   *European Regional Committee*

The Chief Medical Officer was head of the UK delegation to the 44th session of the Regional Committee for Europe, held in Copenhagen in September. Dr Jeremy Metters, Deputy Chief Medical Officer, attended as a member of the Standing Committee of the European Regional Committee. The election for the nomination of the Regional Director from 1995 dominated the first two days of the proceedings. After a ballot, Dr Jo Asvall emerged as the candidate to be put forward to the Executive Board and the World Health Assembly for nomination for a third successive five-year term.

Another major item for discussion was the programme budget for 1996-97: although this budget has only been increased to reflect inflation from the previous biennium (zero-rate growth), it was agreed to try to reduce central costs so as to increase resources for local projects. To achieve this shift, the Committee had to take some difficult decisions about which regular programmes could be demoted in terms of priority: cancer control, medical education and the promotion of research and development, along with reductions in Regional Office support, were identified as areas where savings would be made.

The UK was elected to one of the four seats on WHO's European Environment and Health Committee: subsequently the Chief Medical Officer was nominated as Chairman of this Committee - one of whose objectives is to pave the way for the 3rd European conference on Health and the Environment, which the UK has offered to host in 1999.

The Regional Committee re-affirmed its commitment to working closely with other international organisations such as the European Union and the Council of Europe. The need to avoid duplication and overlap was seen as an increasingly important priority.

(ii)　　*Executive Board*

In January, the Chief Medical Officer attended the 93rd session of the WHO Executive Board in Geneva as the UK's nominated representative. The main item considered was WHO's response to global change. The wide-ranging discussions touched on issues such as the number of terms of office (and their length) to which the Director-General and Regional Directors can be elected, budgetary reform and the future of the Programme Committee.

No decision was made about appointments as there was general agreement that, with no posts to be filled in the near future, time should be taken to allow Member States to reflect on recommendations emerging from the Global Change Working Group. However, there was general support for the establishment of an Administration, Budget and Finance Committee, which would have an important role in reviewing proposals for the budget for the 1996-97 biennium before the Executive Board's considerations in January 1995; it was agreed to complement this Committee with a Programme Development Committee. Together these Committees would take over the duties of the Programme Committee and work closely with the Secretariat, particularly in the key areas of arranging priorities for regular programmes and allocation of resources.

The Executive Board held its second meeting (94th session) in 1994, immediately after the World Health Assembly in May. As the World Health Assembly endorsed the setting up of the two global change sub-committees, the appointment of members to each committee was the most important item of business. The Chief Medical Officer was elected as a member of the Administration, Budget and Finance Committee. The first meetings of both Committees were scheduled for the week immediately before the next Executive Board meeting in January 1995.

(iii)　　*World Health Assembly*

The 47th World Health Assembly, the annual meeting of the Member States of the WHO, took place in Geneva in May. The UK delegation was led by Baroness Cumberlege, Parliamentary Under Secretary of State in the House of Lords, and included the Chief Medical Officer, the Chief Nursing Officer, the UK's Permanent Representative in Geneva and staff from the Mission, and the head of the Health and Population Division of the ODA.

In her address to the plenary session, Baroness Cumberlege spoke of the progress with health reforms in the UK and the development of the Health of the Nation policy[1]. She welcomed WHO's commitment to strengthening nursing and midwifery services and emphasised their important role in promoting health and health care services. Baroness Cumberlege then touched on the importance of ethical issues in health and health care services, not least when it comes to the allocation of resources, underlining the constancy of fundamental ethical principles, even when they were being applied to new challenges.

The Assembly was notable for South Africa's re-admission into full membership of WHO. This was the first UN organisation South Africa had rejoined since its new constitution had come into effect. Another notable event was the announcement by Her Majesty Queen Silvia of Sweden of the establishment of an international foundation dedicated to the prevention of drug abuse among children and adolescents.

Resolutions were passed on action in accordance with recommendations of the Executive Board's Working Group on Global Change, including the setting up of the two sub-Committees - the Administration, Budget and Finance Committee and the Programme Development Committee.

The Assembly passed 32 Resolutions covering a wide range of issues including breast milk substitutes, traditional practices harmful to the health of women and children, and ethical criteria for medicinal drug promotion. The Assembly also passed a Resolution authorising WHO to liaise with other UN Agencies over the setting up of a Joint and Co-sponsored UN programme on HIV/AIDS. This programme will not supersede national programmes but will provide additional support, and represents the first occasion that UN Agencies have been encouraged to co-operate in this way - a clear signal about the need for close and effective international collaboration when dealing with important public health issues. The UN Secretary-General subsequently announced the appointment of Dr Peter Piot in December as leader of this programme.

Reference

1. Department of Health. *The Health of the Nation: a strategy for health in England.* London: HMSO, 1992 (Cm. 1986).

Table A.1: *Population age and sex structure, England, mid-1994, and changes by age, 1981-91, 1991-92, 1992-93 and 1993-94*

Age (in years)	Resident population at mid-1994 (thousands)			Percentage changes (persons)			
	Persons	Males	Females	1981-91	1991-92	1992-93	1993-94
Under 1	634	326	309	10.9	-1.0	-3.6	0.2
1-4	2601	1332	1268	15.2	1.2	0.2	-0.4
5-15	6776	3479	3297	-13.1	1.2	1.8	1.6
16-29	9614	4920	4693	4.7	-2.0	-2.5	-2.5
30-44	10460	5280	5180	11.5	-0.1	0.8	1.5
45-64/59*	9729	5425	4304	-0.2	3.0	2.3	1.8
65/60-74**	5547	1977	3570	-3.2	0.3	0.7	0.5
75-84	2481	926	1555	17.6	-1.3	-2.7	-2.4
85+	864	216	648	49.2	4.7	5.1	3.0
All ages	48707	23882	24825	3.0	0.4	0.3	0.4

* 45-64 years for males and 45-59 years for females.

** 65-74 years for males and 60-74 years for females.

Note: Figures may not add precisely to totals due to rounding.

Source: OPCS

Table A.2: *Five main causes of death for males and females at different ages (and percentages[1] of all causes of deaths), England, 1993*

Rank	All ages - 1 and over		1-14 years		15-34 years		35-54 years		55-74 years		75 years and over	
	Males	Females	Males	Females	Males	Females	Males	Females	Males	Females	Males	Females
1	Ischaemic heart disease	Ischaemic heart disease	Other causes of injury and poisoning†	Diseases of the nervous system	Other causes of injury and poisoning†	Other causes of injury and poisoning†	Ischaemic heart disease	MN* of female breast	Ischaemic heart disease	Ischaemic heart disease	Ischaemic heart disease	Ischaemic heart disease
	29%	22%	17%	15%	22%	15%	26%	19%	33%	23%	27%	24%
2	Cerebro-vascular disease	Cerebro-vascular disease	Diseases of the nervous system	Congenital anomalies	Suicide and self-inflicted injury	Road vehicle accidents	MN* of digestive organs and peritoneum	MN* of genito-urinary organs	MN* of trachea, bronchus and lung	MN* of digestive organs and peritoneum	Pneumonia	Cerebro-vascular disease
	8%	13%	13%	13%	16%	13%	9%	9%	11%	9%	12%	15%
3	MN* of trachea, bronchus and lung	Pneumonia	Road vehicle accidents	Other causes of injury and poisoning†	Road vehicle accidents	Suicide and self-inflicted injury	MN* of trachea, bronchus and lung	MN* of digestive organs and peritoneum	MN* of digestive organs and peritoneum	Cerebro-vascular disease	Cerebro-vascular disease	Pneumonia
	8%	11%	11%	12%	16%	8%	7%	7%	10%	9%	11%	15%
4	Pneumonia	MN* of digestive organs and peritoneum	Congenital anomalies	Road vehicle accidents	Diseases of the nervous system and sense organs	Diseases of the nervous system and sense organs	Other causes of injury and poisoning†	Ischaemic heart disease	Cerebro-vascular disease	MN* of trachea, bronchus and lung	Chronic obstructive pulmonary disease and allied conditions	Diseases of the pulmonary circulation and other forms of heart disease
	8%	6%	9%	9%	5%	7%	6%	7%	6%	8%	8%	7%
5	MN* of digestive organs and peritoneum	Other forms of heart disease	MN* of other and unspecified sites	MN* of other and unspecified sites	Leukaemias	Leukaemias	Suicide and self-inflicted injury	MN* of trachea, bronchus and lung	Chronic obstructive pulmonary disease and allied conditions	MN* of female breast	MN* of digestive organs and peritoneum	MN* of digestive organs and peritoneum
	8%	4%	7%	7%	4%	6%	5%	6%	6%	7%	6%	5%
Remainder	39%	44%	43%	46%	37%	56%	47%	52%	34%	45%	36%	34%
All causes of death	258452	278107	1010	733	5739	2520	17742	11400	104236	70346	129725	193108

[1] May not add up to 100 due to rounding.   * MN = malignant neoplasm.

† 'Other causes of injury and poisoning' comprises categories of external injury and poisoning (E800-E999) excluding road vehicle accidents (E810-E829) and suicide (E950-E959).

Source: OPCS

Table A.3: *Relative mortality from various conditions when presented as numbers of deaths and future years of 'working life' lost, England and Wales, 1993*

Cause (ICD9 code)	Males				Females			
	Number of deaths (thousands)		Years of 'working life' lost (thousands)		Number of deaths (thousands)		Years of 'working life' lost (thousands)	
	All ages	(%)	Age 15-64	(%)	All ages	(%)	Age 15-64	(%)
All causes, all ages	278				298			
All causes, 28 days and over	277	(100)	794	(100)	297	(100)	401	(100)
All malignant neoplasms* (140-208)	74	(27)	176	(22)	67	(22)	181	(45)
Lung cancer (162)	22	(8)	36	(5)	11	(4)	20	(5)
Breast cancer+ (174)					13	(4)	56	(14)
Genito-urinary cancer (179-189)	14	(5)	19	(2)	10	(3)	34	(9)
Leukaemia (204-208)	2	(1)	12	(2)	2	(1)	10	(3)
Circulatory disease* (390-459)	123	(45)	208	(26)	134	(45)	75	(19)
Ischaemic heart disease (410-414)	79	(29)	135	(17)	67	(22)	31	(8)
Cerebrovascular disease (430-438)	23	(8)	26	(3)	38	(13)	24	(6)
Respiratory disease* (460-519)	42	(15)	69	(9)	49	(16)	29	(7)
Pneumonia (480-486)	21	(8)	23	(3)	34	(11)	10	(3)
Bronchitis, emphysema and asthma (490-493)	4	(2)	8	(1)	3	(1)	6	(2)
Sudden infant death syndrome (798.0)	0	(0)	11	(1)	0	(0)	8	(2)
All accidental deaths* (E800-E949)	6	(2)	100	(13)	4	(1)	35	(9)
Motor vehicle traffic accidents (E810-E819)	2	(1)	54	(7)	1	(0)	12	(3)
Suicide (E950-E959)	3	(1)	59	(7)	1	(0)	13	(3)

* These conditions are ranked as well as selected causes within these broader headings. + Not calculated for male breast cancer.

Deaths under 28 days are excluded, except from 'All causes, all ages'. Method of calculation now changed to that set out in DH1 (Mortality Statistics: General: England and Wales).

Source: OPCS

Table A.4: Trends in 'avoidable' deaths, England and Wales, 1979-93. Age-standardised mortality ratios (1979 = 100)

Condition	SMR[1]													Actual number of deaths[4]	
	1979	1982	1983	1984	1985	1986	1987	1988	1989	1990	1991	1992	1993[5]	1979	1993[5]
Hypertension/cerebrovascular (ages 35-64)	100	84	80	77	76	72	68	63	60	57	57*	55	47	9482	4499
Perinatal mortality[2]	100	77	71	69	67	65	61	60	57	55	55	54	61	9400	6033
Cervical cancer (ages 15-64)	100	90	90	91	91	97	89	84	80	77	73	68	63	1142	742
Hodgkin's disease (ages 5-64)	100	86	86	79	75	74	82	74	64	59	57*	59	57	365	231
Respiratory diseases (ages 1-14)	100	87	62	51	50	40	47	40	41	39	41	28	44	329	152
Surgical diseases[3] (ages 5-64)	100	77	71	78	66	72	53	69	52	58	55	60	53	262	138
Asthma (ages 5-44)	100	105	105	102	113	111	111	106	92	84	88	68	37	250	183
Tuberculosis (ages 5-64)	100	91	62	64	65	58	63	55	55	47	47	47	49	222	113
Chronic rheumatic heart disease (ages 5-44)	100	52	42	41	35	34	32	18	26	21	19	14	12	133	22
Total 'avoidable' deaths	100	81	76	74	72	70	66	62	59	57	57	54	49	21585	12113
All causes: ages 0-14 years	100	82	77	73	74	73	72	71	66	62	58	54	51	11132	6052
All causes: ages 15-64 years	100	92	90	88	88	86	84	82	80	78	76	74	72	127194	93097
All causes: all ages	100	94	93	89	92	89	86	85	85	82	82	84	79	591039	576406

[1] The standardised mortality ratio (SMR) for a condition is calculated by dividing the observed number of deaths by the expected number of deaths based on 1979 death rates.

[2] Stillbirths (3,160 in 1993) are included in perinatal mortality and total 'avoidable' deaths, but not in deaths from all causes; the definition of stillbirth changed on 1 October 1992 from a baby born dead after 28 completed weeks gestation to one born dead after 24 weeks gestation.

[3] Appendicitis, abdominal hernia, cholelithiasis and cholecystitis.

[4] Excluding deaths of visitors to England and Wales.

[5] In 1993, changes were made to the way in which deaths were coded to cause; for some causes of death, 1993 data may not be exactly comparable with those for earlier years.

* Revised from figure (58) quoted in 1991 Report.

Source: OPCS

242

Table A.5: *Live births, stillbirths, infant mortality and abortions, England[1], 1960, 1970, 1975-94*

Year	Live births	Stillbirths		Early neonatal mortality (deaths under 1 week)		Perinatal mortality (stillbirths plus deaths under 1 week)	Post-neonatal mortality (deaths 4 weeks to under 1 year)	Infant mortality (deaths under 1 year)	Abortions[1]
	Number	Number	Rate[2]	Number	Rate[3]	Rate[2]	Rate[3]	Rate[3]	Rate[4]
1960	740859	14753	19.5	9772	13.2	32.5	6.3	21.6	-
1970	741999	9708	12.9	7864	10.6	23.4	5.9	18.2	87.6
1975	563900	5918	10.4	5154	9.1	19.4	5.0	15.7	149.9
1976	550393	5339	9.6	4468	8.1	17.6	4.6	14.2	148.7
1977	536953	5087	9.4	4070	7.6	16.9	4.5	13.7	152.7
1978	562589	4791	8.4	3975	7.1	15.4	4.4	13.1	157.7
1979	601316	4811	7.9	4028	6.7	14.6	4.5	12.8	158.8
1980	619371	4523	7.3	3793	6.1	13.4	4.4	12.0	164.5
1981	598163	3939	6.5	3105	5.2	11.7	4.3	10.9	168.8
1982	589711	3731	6.3	2939	5.0	11.2	4.5*	10.8	171.1
1983	593255	3412	5.7	2746	4.6	10.3	4.2	10.0	169.2
1984	600573	3425	5.7	2640	4.4	10.0	3.9	9.4	177.3
1985	619301	3426	5.5	2674	4.3	9.8	3.9	9.2	177.6
1986	623609	3337	5.3	2640	4.2	9.5	4.2	9.5	183.5
1987	643330	3224	5.0	2518	3.9	8.9	4.0	9.1	187.7
1988	654360	3188	4.8	2543	3.9	8.7	4.1	9.1	196.6
1989	649357	3056	4.7	2368	3.6	8.3	3.7	8.4	200.0
1990	666920	3068	4.6	2382	3.6	8.1	3.3	7.9	199.0
1991	660806	3072	4.6	2260	3.4	8.0	3.0	7.3	194.4
1992	651784	2777†	4.2†	2174	3.3	7.6†	2.3	6.5	190.1
1993	636473	3621	5.7	2074	3.3	8.9	2.1	6.3	190.8
1994	628956	3583	5.7	2007	3.2	8.8	2.0	6.1	191.3⁵

[1] Relates to England residents.　[2] Per 1,000 live and stillbirths.　[3] Per 1,000 live births.　[4] Per 1,000 live births, stillbirths and abortions).

[5] Provisional.

* The post-neonatal mortality rate in 1982 has been incorrectly cited as 4.6 per 1,000 live births in some earlier Reports.

† 1992 figures exclude 216 stillbirths of between 24 and 27 completed weeks gestation registered between 1 October 1992 and 31 December 1992, following the introduction of new legislation (see Chapter 1).

Source: OPCS

243

Table A.6: *Congenital malformations, England, 1984, 1990, 1993‡ and 1994†*

ICD Code(s)	Malformation	Live births*				Stillbirths**			
		1984	1990	1993	1994#	1984	1990	1993	1994#
	Malformed babies								
	Number	12812	7520	5292	4351	373	199	147	151
	Rate	213.3	112.8	83.1	69.2	6.2	3.0	2.3	2.4
	Central nervous system								
320-359.9, 740-742.9	Number	597	278	201	155	162	61	42	42
	Rate	9.9	4.2	3.2	2.5	2.7	0.9	0.7	0.7
	Ear and eye								
360-379.9, 743.0-743.9, 744.0-744.3	Number	706	399	218	202	26	12	5	7
	Rate	11.8	6.0	3.4	3.2	0.4	0.2	0.1	0.1
	Cleft lip/cleft palate								
749.0-749.2	Number	796	691	612	497	25	17	8	17
	Rate	13.3	10.4	9.6	7.9	0.4	0.3	0.1	0.3
	Cardiovascular								
390-459.9, 745.0-747.9	Number	775	544	450	344	14	22	17	17
	Rate	12.9	8.2	7.1	5.5	0.2	0.3	0.3	0.3
	Hypospadias/epispadias								
752.6	Number	1082	818	528	455	3	1	-	2
	Rate	18.0	12.3	8.3	7.2	0.0	0.0	-	0.0
	Reduction deformities of limbs								
755.2-755.4	Number	321	188	213	166	13	4	9	7
	Rate	5.3	2.8	3.3	2.6	0.2	0.1	0.1	0.1
	Talipes								
754.5-754.7	Number	1969	998	612	598	22	10	7	7
	Rate	32.8	15.0	9.6	9.5	0.4	0.1	0.1	0.1
	Chromosomal								
758.0-758.9	Number	576	473	372	314	19	21	22	18
	Rate	9.6	7.1	5.8	5.0	0.3	0.3	0.3	0.3

† From January 1990 certain minor malformations are no longer notified, and have been excluded from the figures shown. For example, club foot of positional origin is now excluded from the category 'Talipes', ICD Codes 754.5-754.7. This change in notification practice largely accounts for the decrease in the number of malformations reported in some categories. The format of this table also differs from that in previous years to reflect ICD changes.

* Rates per 10,000 live births. ** Rates per 10,000 total births. # Provisional data; rates for 1993 are not available.

Source: OPCS

Table A.7: *Cancer* registrations by age and site, males, England and Wales, 1990*

	Numbers and percentages															
	Age-group (years)															
	All ages		0-14 years		15-24 years		25-44 years		45-64 years		65-74 years		75-84 years		85 years and over	
		%		%		%		%		%		%		%		%
Eye, brain and other nervous system	2111	2	163	22	79	9	329	7	860	3	480	1	181	1	19	0
Mouth and pharynx	2062	2	6	1	16	2	154	3	835	3	622	2	344	1	85	1
Oesophagus	3044	3	0	0	0	0	60	1	884	3	1106	3	824	3	170	2
Lung	25151	24	1	0	7	1	309	7	6443	25	9738	28	7283	24	1370	20
Stomach	6472	6	1	0	5	1	113	3	1521	6	2324	7	2023	7	485	7
Pancreas	3040	3	0	0	0	0	54	1	848	3	981	3	956	3	201	3
Large intestine and rectum	13922	13	5	1	13	2	352	8	3673	14	4623	13	4199	14	1057	15
Prostate	13481	13	3	0	2	0	15	0	1639	6	4512	13	5771	19	1539	22
Bladder	8214	8	2	0	6	1	176	4	2099	8	2840	8	2425	8	666	10
Skin (melanoma)†	1467	1	5	1	45	5	335	7	542	2	294	1	202	1	44	1
Leukaemias and lymphomas	8010	8	330	45	302	36	906	20	2167	8	2090	6	1779	6	436	6
All other cancer	16698	16	222	30	358	43	1684	38	4730	18	4899	14	3877	13	928	13
Total cancer	103672	100	738	100	833	100	4487	100	26241	100	34509	100	29864	100	7000	100

* Cancer = malignant neoplasm.
† Melanoma of skin only (ICD9 code 172). Earlier reports included figures for other malignant neoplasm of skin (ICD9 code 173), which are greatly under-registered.

Note: Percentages may not add up to 100 due to rounding.

Source: OPCS

245

Table A.8: Cancer* registrations by age and site, females, England and Wales, 1990

Numbers and percentages

Age-group (years)

	All ages	%	0-14 years	%	15-24 years	%	25-44 years	%	45-64 years	%	65-74 years	%	75-84 years	%	85 years and over	%
Eye, brain and other nervous system	1647	2	130	23	65	9	242	3	595	2	368	1	204	1	43	0
Mouth and pharynx	1229	1	5	1	13	2	89	1	356	1	344	1	288	1	134	1
Oesophagus	2213	2	0	0	0	0	17	0	373	1	597	2	840	3	386	3
Breast	28812	27	3	1	27	4	3247	39	12349	39	6276	23	4860	18	2050	19
Lung	11612	11	0	0	8	1	212	3	3071	10	4308	16	3206	12	807	7
Stomach	4025	4	1	0	3	0	73	1	545	2	998	4	1603	6	802	7
Pancreas	3215	3	0	0	3	0	33	0	598	2	942	3	1161	4	478	4
Large intestine and rectum	13790	13	0	0	10	1	331	4	2775	9	3743	14	4673	18	2258	20
Ovary	5065	5	10	2	44	6	440	5	1918	6	1380	5	957	4	316	3
Cervix	4310	4	0	0	54	8	1588	19	1416	5	720	3	406	2	126	1
Other uterus	4156	4	0	0	2	0	160	2	1684	5	1138	4	864	3	308	3
Bladder	3176	3	2	0	6	1	62	1	601	2	905	3	1111	4	489	4
Skin (melanoma)†	2155	2	4	1	93	13	517	6	716	2	369	1	312	1	144	1
Leukaemias and lymphomas	6678	6	245	43	218	32	557	7	1504	5	1643	6	1756	7	755	7
All other cancer	13659	13	166	29	143	21	772	9	2906	9	3542	13	4181	16	1949	18
Total cancer	105742	100	566	100	689	100	8340	100	31407	100	27273	100	26422	100	11045	100

* Cancer = malignant neoplasm.

† Melanoma of skin only (ICD9 code 172). Earlier reports included figures for other malignant neoplasm of skin (ICD9 code 173), which are greatly under-registered.

Note: Percentages may not add up to 100 due to rounding.

Source: OPCS

Table A.9: *Percentage of children immunised by their 2nd birthday and of children given BCG vaccine by their 14th birthday, England, 1980-93/94*

Year	Diphtheria	Tetanus	Polio	Whooping cough	Measles	Mumps/ rubella	BCG[1]
1980[2]	81	81	81	41	53	-	82
1981[2]	83	83	82	46	55	-	78
1982[2]	84	84	84	53	58	-	75
1983[2]	84	84	84	59	60	-	76
1984[2]	84	84	84	65	63	-	71
1985[2]	85	85	85	65	68	-	77
1986[2]	85	85	85	67	71	-	76
1987/88[2]	87	87	87	73	76	-	76
1988/89	87	87	87	75	80	7	71
1989/90	89	89	89	78	84	68	36[3]
1990/91	92	92	92	84	87	86	90[3]
1991/92	93	93	93	88	90	90	86[3]
1992/93	95	95	95	92	92	92	74
1993/94	95	95	95	93	91	91	79

1 Estimated percentage.

2 Estimated percentage immunised by the end of the second year after birth.

3 The school BCG programme was suspended in 1989 because there were insufficient supplies of BCG vaccine; figures for the subsequent two years were relatively higher as a result.

Sources: 1980-87/88: Form SBL 607
1988/89 onwards: Form KC51 (except BCG); KC50 (BCG)

Table A.10: *Cumulative totals of AIDS cases by exposure category, England, to 31 December 1994*

(Numbers subject to revision as further data are received or duplicates identified)

How persons probably acquired the virus	Number of cases			
	Male	Female	Total	%+
Sexual intercourse:				
Between men	7095	-	7095	75
Between men and women				
'High risk' partner*	31	82	113	1
Other partner abroad**	553	378	931	10
Other partner UK	54	41	95	1
Partner's risk not known	15	3	18	<1
Injecting drug use (IDU)	255	111	366	4
IDU and sexual intercourse				
between men	154	-	154	2
Blood				
Blood factor (eg haemophiliacs)	407	5	412	4
Blood or tissue transfer (eg transfusion)				
Abroad	12	40	52	1
UK	19	21	40	<1
Mother to child	67	68	135	1
Other/undetermined	83	16	99	1
Total	8145	765	9510	100

* Includes men and women who had sex with injecting drug users, or with those infected through blood factor treatment or blood transfusion, and women who had sex with bisexual men.

** Includes persons without other identified risks who are from, or who have lived in, countries where the major route of HIV-1 transmission is through sexual intercourse between men and women.

+ Total does not add up to 100 because of rounding.

Source: CDSC

Table A.11: *Expectation of life at birth, all-cause death rates and infant mortality, England and European Community countries, circa 1992*

Country	Year	Expection of life at birth		All cause mortality rate*		Infant mortality rate**
		Men	Women	Men	Women	
England	1992	73.9†	79.5†	299.7	180.2	6.5
United Kingdom	1992	73.5	79.2	312.7	187.2	6.6
Belgium	1989	72.3	79.1	353.4	184.2	8.5
Denmark	1992	72.7	78.2	361.0	228.9	6.5
Germany	1991	72.3	78.9	382.3	184.3	6.9
Greece	1991	74.7	80.1	299.2	138.8	9.0
France	1991	73.5	82.0	379.4	154.1	7.3
Ireland	1991	72.2	77.9	346.3	194.4	7.6
Italy	1990	73.7	80.5	322.9	150.4	8.0
Luxembourg	1992	72.6	79.3	357.2	183.4	7.2
Netherlands	1992	74.3	80.5	282.9	164.8	6.3
Portugal	1993	70.6	77.9	432.0	192.7	8.7
Spain	1991	73.4	80.7	347.3	144.0	7.2
EC average	*1991*	*73.1*	*79.9*	*352.8*	*169.7*	*7.5*

* Per 100,000 population aged 0-64 years, age-standardised using the WHO 'old' European standard population.

**Per 1,000 live births.

† Figure for England and Wales, calculated by WHO, presented for comparability with other international data; equivalent figures calculated by slightly different methodology by the Government Actuary's Department are 73.8 years for men and 79.2 years for women.

Source: WHO European Office 'Health for All' statistical database

Figure A1: *Weekly deaths, England and Wales, 1993 and 1994, and expected deaths, 1994*

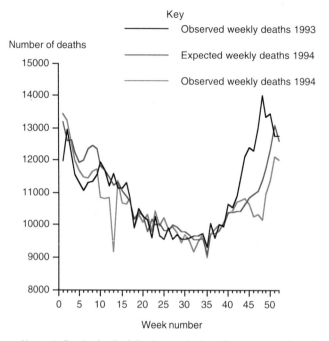

Key

——— Observed weekly deaths 1993

——— Expected weekly deaths 1994

——— Observed weekly deaths 1994

Notes: i. Deaths for the following weeks have been averaged to take account of the Easter and Christmas holidays: weeks 1992/51, 52, 53 and 1993/1; weeks 1993/14 and 15; weeks 1993/52 and 1994/1, and weeks 1994/13 and 14.
ii. Data are for 1-year-olds and over.

Source: OPCS

Printed in the United Kingdom for HMSO
Dd 301075 C40 9/95 13110